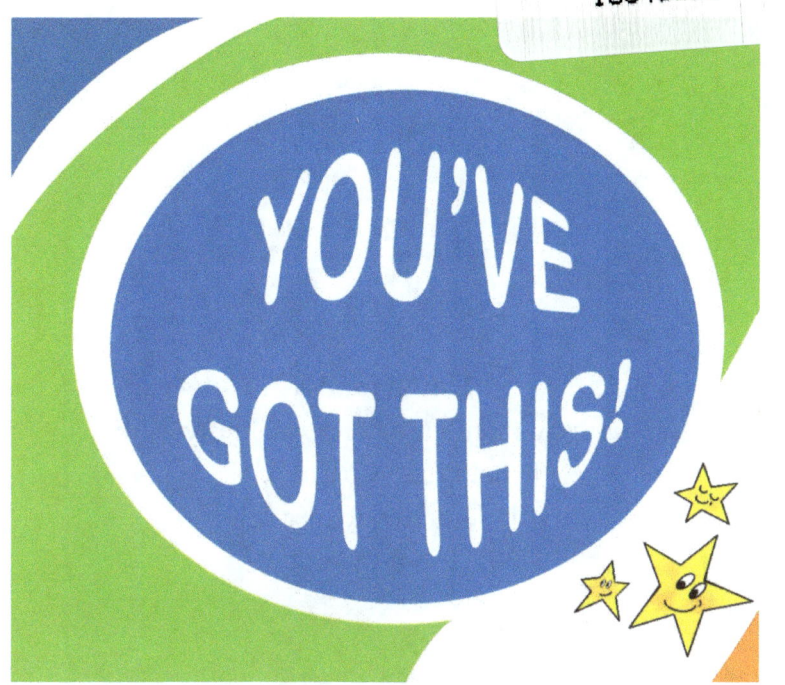

Also by the Authors

Eating for A's
A month-by-month nutrition and lifestyle guide
to help raise smarter kids
(Kindergarten to 6th grade)
ISBN 978-0-9848540-0-4

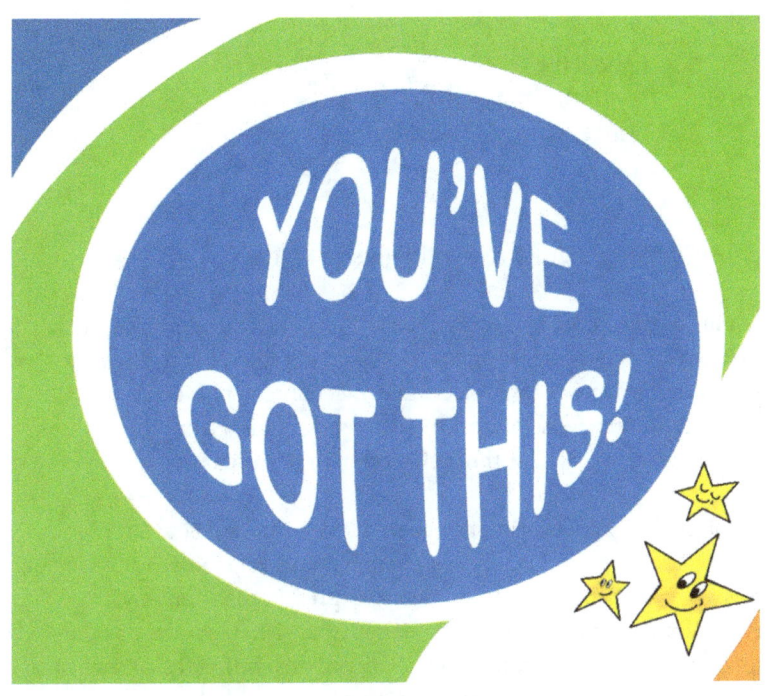

**45 Doable Tips for Teens to
Feel Good, Look Good & Succeed**

Lorna A. Williams, MPH, RD
Kathleen M. Dunn, MPH, RD

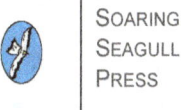 SOARING
SEAGULL
PRESS

You've Got This!
45 Doable Tips for Teens to Feel Good, Look Good & Succeed

 Published by:
Soaring Seagull Press
Santa Rosa, CA 95401
EatingFor.com

© 2023 Soaring Seagull Press. All rights reserved.

No part of this book, including interior design, cover design and illustrations may be reproduced, stored in a retrieval system or transmitted by any means, electronic, mechanical, photocopying, recording or otherwise, without written permission from the authors and publisher, except for the inclusion of brief quotations in a review.

Although every precaution has been taken in the preparation of this book, the authors and publisher assume no responsibility for errors or omissions. The authors and publisher expressly disclaim any responsibility for any liability, loss, injury or risk, personal or otherwise, which is incurred as a consequence, directly or indirectly, of the use and application of any of the contents of this book.

The information in this book is provided for educational purposes and general reference. It is not meant to be a substitute for medical advice or counseling. Consult a physician before making any changes to diet, exercise or other health habits as described in this book.

All trademarks are the property of their respective owners.

ISBN: 978-0-9848540-1-1
Library of Congress Control Number: 2022946360

Cover Design and Artwork by Lorna A. Williams

Printed in the United States of America

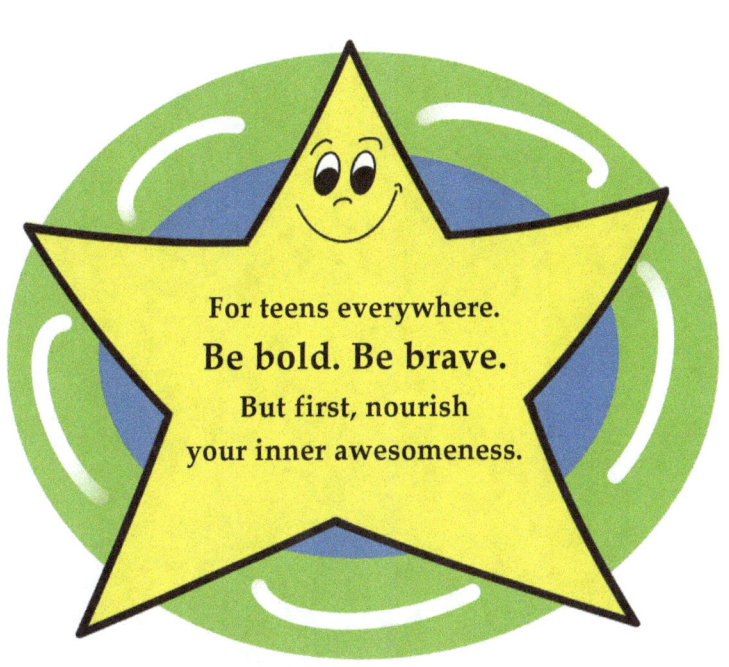

Contents

Start Here 1

15 Tips to Feel Good 5

1. For good grades and an active social life, turn to the power of sleep. 6
2. For peak performance during the day, improve your sleep habits. 8
3. To knock stress down to size, think balance. 10
4. To relax, make time to reflect. 12
5. To stay in the stress-free zone, say hello to yoga. 14
6. To help banish test anxiety, get enough vitamin C. 16
7. To fuel your body (and brain), fill your plate with veggies and fruits. 18
8. To get more from plant foods, eat a variety in a rainbow of colors. 20
9. For a phytonutrient payload, eat more salads. 22
10. To detoxify and fortify your health, eat more cruciferous veggies. 24
11. To brighten up a meal, add a colorful grain. 26
12. To get more from life, take time to taste. 28
13. To encourage a friend, send inspiring text messages. 30
14. For better heart health, volunteer to help others. 32
15. For a happier day, move more. 34

15 Tips to Look Good 37

1. To put your best face forward, eat more carotenoid-rich veggies and fruits. 38
2. For a clear skin routine that really works, fill your plate with low-GI foods. 40
3. To soothe dry, itchy winter skin, get enough vitamin D. 42
4. To control acne severity, consume more skin-friendly fats. 44
5. To fight acne, turn to the power of vitamin A. 46
6. To smile bright, fine-tune your food choices and eating habits. 48
7. To protect your dazzling smile, pick the right kind of gum. 50
8. To protect your pearly whites, lighten up on sports and energy drinks. 52
9. To avoid eye strain, fill your plate with lutein-rich foods and take blinking breaks. 54
10. To unleash your growth potential, get enough calcium. 56
11. For stronger bones, know all the nutrients that matter. 58
12. To instantly look better, stand tall. 60
13. For muscle building, eat enough protein. 62
14. For muscle building, choose protein foods rich in leucine. 64
15. For muscle building, eat protein foods at the right time. 66

15 Tips to Succeed 69
1. To be your best, fill your plate for performance.......... 70
2. To feel full and satisfied, eat enough fiber. 72
3. To make sure you're fully hydrated, take a look at your pee. 74
4. To control inflammation, say goodbye to added sugars. 76
5. To be ready for early morning zero periods, prepare the no-brainer way. 78
6. For benefits that last all day, eat a high-protein breakfast. 80
7. To banish caffeine jitters, find your Goldilocks balance. 82
8. For better test scores, fine-tune how you eat................ 84
9. For strong immunity, start with what you eat............. 86
10. To fully enjoy your winter adventures, fortify your immune health... 88
11. To be healthier, happier and more successful, try the mealtime secret. 90
12. To lower your pesticide burden, choose cleaner vegetables and fruits... 92
13. For an easier way to shape new habits, be like bamboo. 94
14. Follow your taste buds, and your future self will thank you. 96
15. To fill nutrient gaps, take a daily multivitamin............ 98

Nutrition Resources & Quick Meal Ideas 101
    Stretch Your gRAINBOW 102
    Carotenoid-rich Foods for Healthy Looking Skin 108
    Key Bone-building Nutrients 110
    Where's the Protein? 112
    Where's the Leucine? 114
    Where's the Fiber? 116
    Power Smoothie Recipes 120
    Caffeine by the Numbers 124
    Breakfast in Under 5 Minutes 126

Acknowledgements 129
About the Authors 129
References 130
Index 136

Start Here

Get ready to feel good, look good and be more successful by tapping into one of the most overlooked and underappreciated actions you can take. You'll find this superpower hiding in plain sight in the diet and lifestyle choices you make every day. You just need to focus on the right ones. Choices like brushing your teeth, drinking enough water or eating vegetables. Sounds simple, right? It is, but it's far from easy, until now.

In the pages that follow, you'll find 45 tips just for teens to make it easier to choose the habits that matter. You'll learn why these specific habits are important (and the research behind them). You'll also find plenty of suggestions to help you add them to your regular routine (without taxing your brain or emptying your wallet).

Shaping habits takes practice, but if you stick with it, you'll soon build a momentum that's tough to slow down. In this way, you'll be turning small, doable actions into healthy habits that last a lifetime. Think of it as training for the ultimate goal: To fortify your ability to be calm and resilient, refreshed and energized, and ready to face any day with confidence.

Pick a tip, track your progress, get to your goals

How can you best use the information in this book? That depends on you. You may be a methodical type and prefer to start at the beginning. That's great. Or, you may prefer to flip through the pages to find a tip that appeals to you to work on first. That's great, too. Either way works, you just need to pick one and get started.

A closer look at the categories

The Feel Good category (the green stamps) is the first category. Here, you'll find 15 tips to help you build habits to sleep better, destress and nourish your inner champion, so you can blast through your day, yet stay calm, cool and collected.

The Look Good category (the orange stamps) is next. Here, you'll find 15 tips to help you fight acne, unleash your growth potential, protect your smile and more, so you can blaze your own trail with confidence.

Finally, the Succeed category (the blue stamps) includes 15 tips to make it easier for you to fuel your body, feed your brain and level up your mindset, so you can seriously excel in school (and in life).

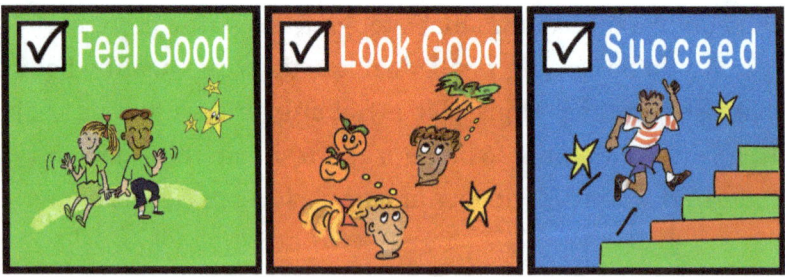

Aim to work on one tip each week

Your best strategy is to pick one tip to focus on each week. Schedule the same day of the week, say each Sunday, to decide on the tip you'll work on for that week (this helps make tracking your progress easier). Some tips like getting the right amount of sleep may take longer to become a solid habit. That's OK. Keep at it for another week or so and, once you feel confident it's part of your routine, check off the corresponding stamp and move on to another tip.

As you flip through the book, you may find some tips you already do and others that may not apply to you. Check those off as well. In addition, each section starts with a complete set of 15 stamps. Check those off too as you make progress and enjoy the boost of confidence that comes with mastery.

Go ahead, put pen (or pencil) to paper and check away, make notes and scribble about what works (and what doesn't). In other words, mark up the book as you please. Why? The act of writing by hand or even doodling activates deep learning that helps you make progress. To help, you'll find space to write notes at the end of each tip and at the end of each section.

Be sure to keep this book in plain sight, on your night stand, at your desk, anywhere that will make it easy to grab when you're ready to track your progress. Remember, it's all about building a mindset for mastery, and tracking your progress is one of the fastest ways to get there.

Understand the techy talk

While we've avoided technical terms that only nutrition scientists seem to love, we did include two somewhat techy terms that may need defining. The first term is "antioxidant." Antioxidants are compounds that help neutralize harmful free radicals that routinely form in the body as a result of a variety of lifestyle factors. One factor is being overweight, others include smoking, sun exposure, pollution and even something beneficial like exercise. When your body is overwhelmed by these unstable molecules, they can do all sorts of damage to your cells and tissues. Even your DNA or genetic material can be damaged by an excess production of free radicals. For this reason, you may want to pay extra attention to tips that help you consume more antioxidant-rich foods like vegetables and fruits. The second term is "phytonutrient." *Phyto* is Greek for plant, and nutrient means any substance that nourishes the body. So, phytonutrients are plant-based compounds that have health benefits.

Celebrate progress, not perfection

Keep in mind that developing a healthy habit isn't about being perfect. Rather, it's about making progress, little by little, day by day, until a habit becomes second nature.

One final reminder. If you think you need to rush forward, think again. This is not a race. Rather, it's a journey that moves you one step closer to being your best you. So, go at your own pace and enjoy the journey. After all, you're building healthy habits that not only help you succeed during your teen years, but ones that help unleash your full potential at every age.

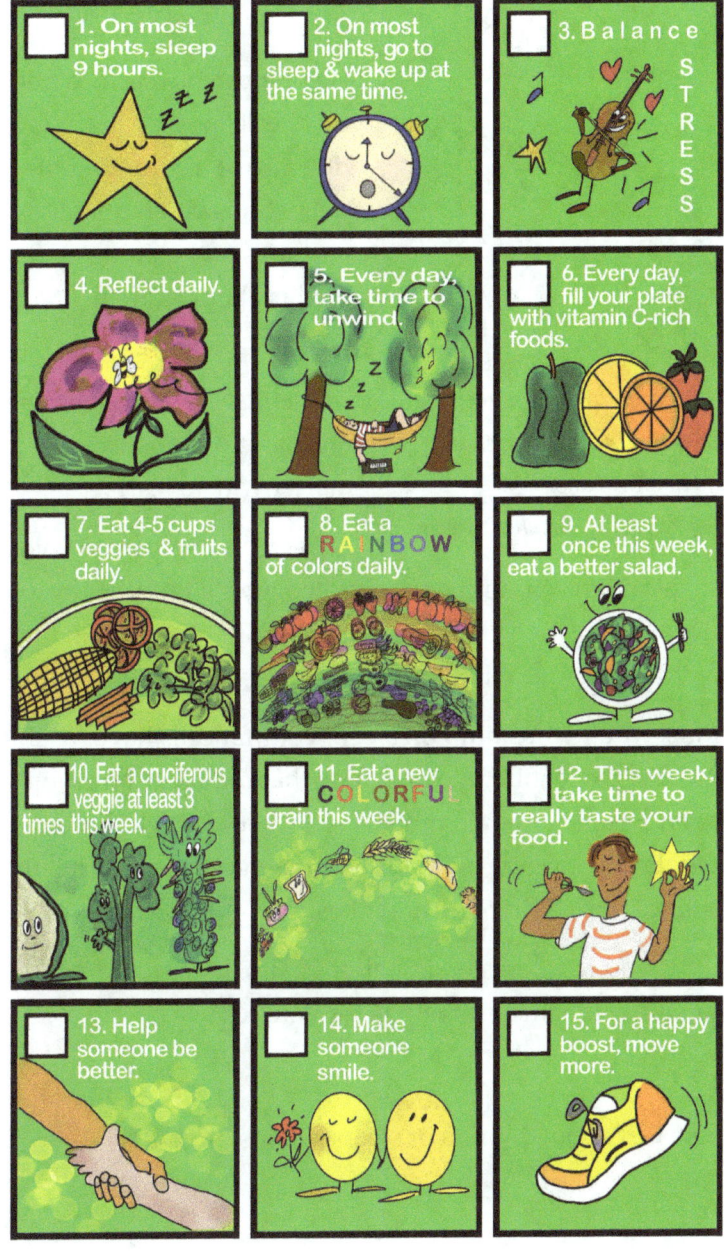

1 For good grades and an active social life, turn to the power of sleep.

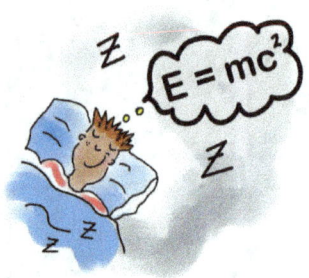

A good laugh and a long sleep are the best cures in the doctor's book.
—Irish Proverb

Sleep helps you learn. While you're asleep, your brain is wide awake, processing the day's events, strengthening memories and gaining new insights about learned activities.

Scientists call this memory consolidation. You can call it a smarter way to learn.

Sleep also helps you enjoy your social life. Without enough sleep, you'll muddle through your day in a groggy haze. This makes it harder for you to enjoy fun activities with your friends.

Plus, when you skimp on sleep, your fat cells have trouble responding to insulin, the hormone that regulates how you store and use energy.[1] In other words, your fat cells become metabolically groggy, and you become more prone to insulin resistance, type 2 diabetes and obesity.[2]

So, if you're interested in better health, better grades and a better social life, then this tip is for you.

■ ■ ■

To Do: Get about 9 hours of sleep on most nights.

3 ways to get enough sleep

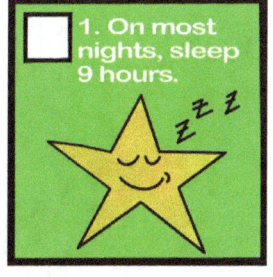

You need between 8 and 10 hours of sleep each night.[3] Yet, most teens get only about 6½ hours of nightly slumber. If this sounds like you, check out these simple ways to get more restful sleep:

1 **Reduce overstimulation.** Avoid energy drinks, coffee and other caffeine-containing drinks at least 3 to 5 hours before bedtime. This helps give your liver time to metabolize caffeine so it's less likely to disrupt your sleep.

2 **Activate your sleep hormone.** Avoid using a smartphone, computer or other device that emits artificial blue light a few hours before bedtime. These screens suppress the brain's production of melatonin, the hormone that helps you fall asleep.

3 **Unwind from your day.** Enjoy a soothing cup of chamomile tea before bedtime. This calming herb has a history of traditional use that hails back to the ancient Egyptians, Romans and Greeks. It remains popular today because, well, it works.

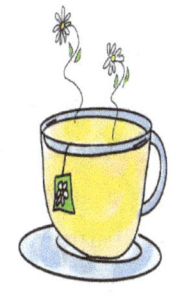

Are you getting enough Zzz's. If not, what can you do?

Notes: _____

_____

_____

> ### 2   For peak performance during the day, improve your sleep habits.

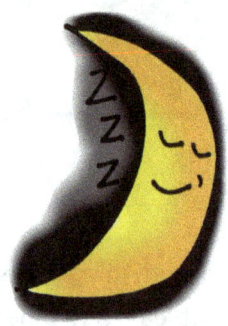

Sleep is the single most effective thing we can do to reset our brain and body health each day.
—Mathew Walker

In the previous tip, you learned why getting enough sleep is so important, but it's equally important to have a regular sleep schedule.

Scientists have yet to confirm the real reason we need sleep, but they do know one thing: Regular sleep benefits all body functions. Yes, all of them.

Even one day without enough sleep can spell trouble beyond the expected daytime grogginess, not to mention the inability to concentrate on tasks.[4]

Consider what happens in areas with Daylight Savings Time. In the spring when people turn their clocks forward, they lose one hour of possible sleep. The next day, a spike in heart attacks has been shown to occur. The opposite occurs in the autumn when clocks are turned back and people gain an additional hour for restful sleep.[5] In other words, even a minor change in your sleep routine can profoundly affect how you function during the day.

■ ■ ■

To Do: On most nights, go to sleep and wake up at the same time.

4 tips for a better sleep routine

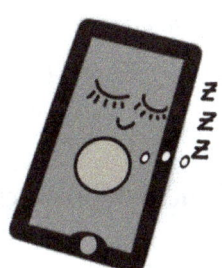

1. **Keep a regular schedule.** Even on weekends, go to sleep and wake up at regular times. This helps you stay in tune with your body's natural circadian rhythm and maintain peak mental and physical performance. It can help to have a "lights out" policy, say from 9:30 p.m. to 6:30 a.m.

2. **Think comfort.** Make sure your bedroom has the three critical elements (cool, dark and quiet) you need to comfortably fall asleep and stay asleep.

3. **Set your phone to wind down mode.** Most smart phones have a wind down mode that helps reduce distraction before bedtime so you can relax and fall asleep.

4. **Rise and shine, naturally.** If you have trouble getting up in the dark morning hours, check out some of the sunrise alarm clocks designed to help you wake up naturally by mimicking dawn's early light.

How are your sleep patterns? Keep track below.

Notes: _____
_____
_____

3   To knock stress down to size, think balance.

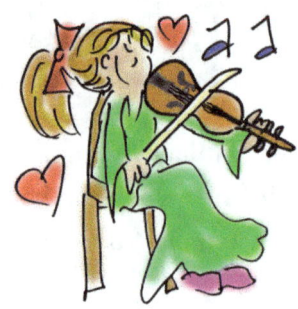

Stress is a balancing act.
Too much = burnout.
Too little = boredom.
In the middle is where you find your superpowers.
           —Allison Graham

If you're like many busy teens, you may feel like you're under too much stress.

Even the toughest teen can crack under a schedule that starts with an early morning zero period or is packed with activities into the evening hours.

The good news is you can make stress work for you. It's all about balance.

While you need some stress to get moving and be productive, too much can put you on overload. It's like the strings on a violin. Too loose, and the music moans and groans. Too tight, and the music shrieks. Only the right amount of tension produces beautiful music.

It's the same with stress. When you balance your stress level, you're better prepared to excel in school and in life.

Now, that's the sound of beautiful music.

■ ■ ■

To Do: Every day, do something to balance stress.

4 stress-busters for better balance

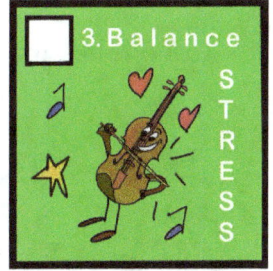

If you want to stay calm and focused throughout your day, check out these four stress-busters you can put into practice right now:

1 **Balance school, play, family and friendships.** Like a violin with four strings, you need all four areas of your life in balance so you can flourish.

2 **Use a daily planner.** Writing down all the things on your schedule (including homework assignments) can help you better manage your time and relieve stress.

3 **Break big projects into smaller chunks.** To manage a project that feels overwhelming, break it down into smaller tasks and chip away at it on a regular basis. In this way, you're more likely to deliver your project on time without losing sleep or feeling too stressed.

4 **Surround yourself with a favorite scent.** How about lavender, citrus or coconut? You'll breathe deeper, which helps lower your heart rate and blood pressure.

What can you do to manage your stress?

Notes: _____
_____
_____

4   To relax, make time to reflect.

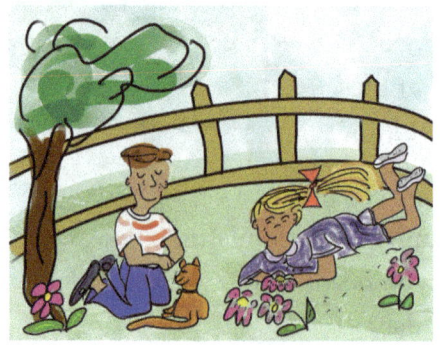

Even if you do things you're passionate about like soccer, dance, music or theater, doing too much without enough rest can leave you feeling physically drained, unable to focus and just plain sap your spirit.

There's one way to help banish that pressure-cooker feeling. It's free, easy and only takes a few minutes.

Here it is: Take a few minutes to stop what you're doing and just look at and listen to the world around you. It may seem counter-intuitive, but this one habit can bring calm to the rest of your day. Really, it's that simple.

Don't Just

Don't just learn, experience.
Don't just read, absorb.
Don't just change, transform.
Don't just relate, advocate.
Don't just promise, prove.
Don't just criticize, encourage.
Don't just think, ponder.
Don't just take, give.
Don't just see, feel.
Don't just dream, do.
Don't just hear, listen.
Don't just talk, act.
Don't just tell, show.
Don't just exist, live.
                —Roy T. Bennett

■ ■ ■

To Do: Take 5 minutes every day to look, listen and learn.

Start here for calmer days

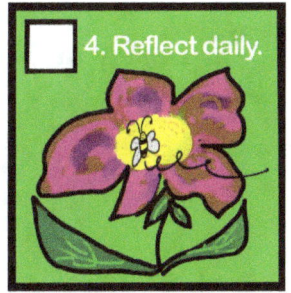

Taking time each day to slow down, even just a little bit, can help bring calm to the rest of your day, help you be more productive and ultimately be your best you. This is an often-overlooked trick that can deliver huge benefits when you're feeling stressed out.

Here's how to get started. First, set aside 15 minutes each day to just observe the world around you. If this feels like FOREVER, that's OK. Start with a shorter length of time, say 5 minutes, and build up from there.

Next, breathe deeply as you take in the sights around you and the sounds that fill the air. Breathe in slowly through your nose and out through your mouth. (Place your hand on your belly, and if it expands when you inhale, you know you're breathing deeply.)

Take it all in, quietly and with intention. Make this a daily habit, and you'll likely feel calmer throughout the day. Even better, this mindful practice can help you feel more resilient and capable of overcoming the obstacles keeping you from your goals. In other words, it's a simple habit with serious benefits for your emotional wellbeing.

Notes: _____
_____
_____

5   To stay in the stress-free zone, say hello to yoga.

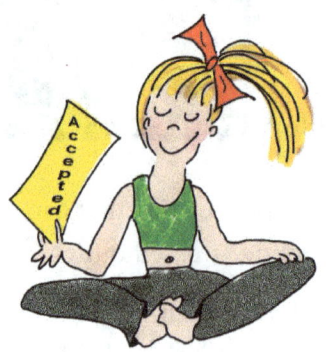

Sometimes the most important thing in a whole day is the rest we take between two deep breaths.
—Etty Hittlesum

If school has you feeling overwhelmed, maybe it's time to try Kripalu-style yoga. High school juniors and seniors who practice this style of yoga have a better mood and less tension and anxiety, according to one Harvard study.[6] That's powerful stuff from simple yoga poses, breathing exercises, and a few daily moments of relaxation and meditation.

How does it work? Researchers attribute the happy effect of Kripalu-style yoga to its ability to boost the brain's level of gamma-aminobutyric acid (GABA), a key biochemical messenger involved in mood and anxiety.

Adding Kripalu yoga to your routine may be just what you need to stay positive and in the stress-free zone. In this way, you can more easily navigate whatever comes your way, including the nail-biting wait for college acceptance letters to roll in. It's not magic, but it may be the next best thing.

■ ■ ■

To Do: Every day, take time to unwind

Calm relaxation starts here

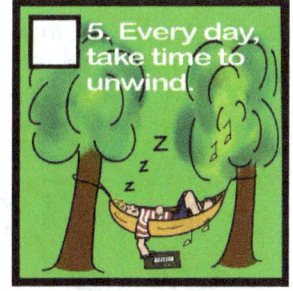

1. **Say yes to yoga.** Kripalu yoga may help you have a more relaxed, positive attitude. Learn more at the Kripalu Center for Yoga & Health (kripalu.org). You'll even find free (yes, free) online options for at-home or on-the-go relaxation techniques like watching 1-hour, at-home yoga classes or listening to quick, 5-minute yoga breaks.

2. **Choose foods rich in vitamin B6.** Vitamin B6 is a cofactor for the brain's production of GABA and other biochemical messengers that help regulate your mood. Good food sources include animal-based foods like meat, fish, eggs and dairy products and plant-based foods like whole grain cereals, vegetables, dried beans and some fruits.

3. **Take a daily multi.** A high-quality multivitamin can help fill nutrient gaps between what your diet provides and what your brain needs for optimal GABA production.

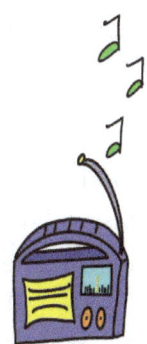

Notes: _____
_____
_____

6   To help banish test anxiety, get enough vitamin C.

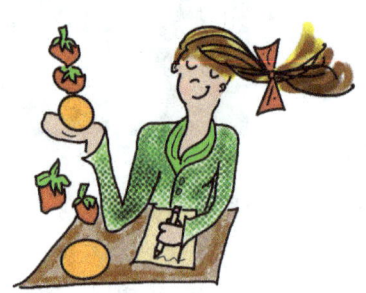

When anxiety is looming, it's tough to perform at your best. If you're feeling anxious, a calmer state of mind could be as simple as getting enough vitamin C, according to one study.[7]

Everybody is a genius. But if you judge a fish by its ability to climb a tree, it will spend its whole life believing that it is stupid.
—Albert Einstein

For this study, researchers randomly assigned 42 moderately anxious, but otherwise healthy, high school students to one of two treatments: a vitamin C supplement (500 milligrams per day) or a dummy pill (placebo). Compared to the placebo group, the vitamin C group significantly reduced their anxiety level after only two weeks.

The researchers believe vitamin C helps reduce oxidative stress in the brain, which is associated with anxiety. Vitamin C may also modulate the action of neurotransmitters, the biochemical messengers nerve cells use to communicate. In fact, the central role of vitamin C in the synthesis of neurotransmitters likely explains its high level in the brain.

■ ■ ■

To Do: Every day, fill your plate with vitamin-C rich foods.

Fill your plate with calm

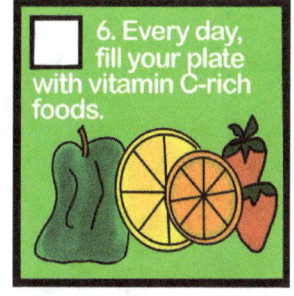

How do you get the same amount of anxiety-reducing vitamin C on your daily plate? You could take a daily supplement with 500 milligrams like the students in the study did. (Check your multivitamin; it just may meet the mark.)

You could also eat more vitamin C-rich foods. Think fresh vegetables and fruits, especially citrus fruits. Here are a few ideas to get you started, each providing about 100 milligrams of vitamin C per serving:

- For a grab-and-go snack, reach for an orange (1 large)
- Top off a lunch salad with sweet red pepper strips (1/2 cup)
- Serve up steamed broccoli at dinner (1 cup)
- For a sweet treat, grab some fresh strawberries (1 cup)
- For a tropical twist, enjoy a bowl of fresh pineapple chunks (1¼ cup)

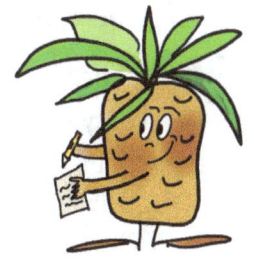

Notes: _____
_____
_____

> **7** **To fuel your body (and brain), fill your plate with veggies and fruits.**

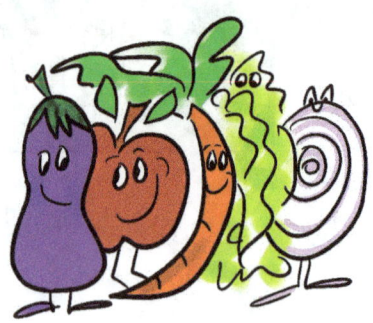

People who love to eat are always the best people.
—*Julia Child*

Vegetables and fruits provide nutrients that nourish and protect your body and brain, you just need to eat enough of them.

Think essential vitamins, minerals and other health-promoting plant compounds (phytonutrients).

Continue this habit into adulthood, and you'll increase your odds of staying healthy, year after year.

It's no surprise that a healthful diet is a plant-based diet. After all, the amazing ways plant compounds impact health is an active area of research. Yet, a nationwide survey[8] of more than 13,300 high school students reveals only 7% eat enough fruit and, worse, only 2% eat enough veggies.

You can buck this dismal trend by following one simple rule: Eat plenty of vegetables and fruits throughout your day (including at breakfast and snack time).

■ ■ ■

To Do: Eat 4 to 5 cups of veggies and fruits every day.

An easy way to fill your plate

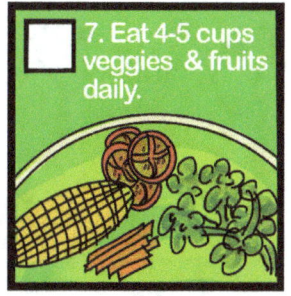

You may be surprised to learn you only need a few servings of vegetables and fruit every day to help fully nourish your body.

In fact, it could be as little as four cups, according to the current Dietary Guidelines for Americans (2020-2025).[9] Here's the minimum intake recommended for teens:

- **Teen Girls**
  Vegetables: At least 2½ cups per day
  Fruits: At least 1½ cups per day

- **Teen Boys**
  Vegetables: At least 3 cups per day
  Fruits: At least 2 cups per day

These guidelines are for moderately active teens (those who get about 30 minutes of exercise beyond normal daily activities). If you're more active, you'll want to eat more, especially more veggies.

For more inspiration on how to boost your intake of vegetables and fruits, check out the tips at www.myplate.gov.

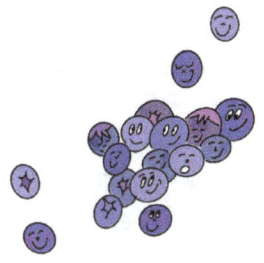

Notes:
_____
_____
_____

| 8 | **To get more from plant foods, eat a variety in a rainbow of colors.** |

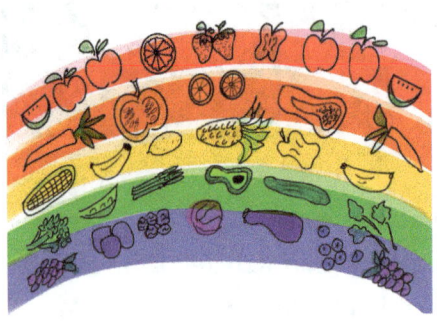

Eat the colors of the rainbow.
— *Anonymous*

Your body benefits from the same naturally occurring compounds that protect plants from pollution, predators, diseases and other threats.

Scientists call these compounds phytonutrients. They number in the thousands and give the plant foods you eat their color, aroma and flavor. But here's the rub: The phytonutrient profile of a lemon, orange or other citrus fruit is different than that of broccoli and other cruciferous vegetables. Likewise, a red tomato has a different phytonutrient profile than an orange carrot or a purple plum. What's more, each phytonutrient profile exerts different health benefits.

For this reason, you'll want to eat a wide variety of vegetables and fruits in all the color groups. In this way, you can get the most out of the phytonutrients in plant foods.

In other words, variety matters, but so does color, especially if you want to level up the protective power of the plant foods you eat.

■ ■ ■

To Do: Every day, eat a variety of vegetables and fruits in a rainbow of colors.

3 ways to get more phytonutrients

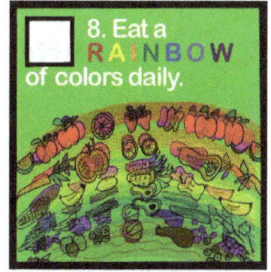

You can take the drama out of fueling your body with as many protective phytonutrients as possible when you follow these three basic guidelines:

1 **Add variety to your menu.** The next time you're at the grocery store, check out the produce section. You'll find vegetables and fruits that you recognize, but look closer and you'll likely find new ones just waiting for you to try.

2 **Expand your color palette.** Vegetables and fruits fall into five color groups: red, yellow/orange, green, purple/blue and white/tan. Make it a game and see how many different colors you can eat at each meal.

3 **Look for inspiration.** For fun facts and ideas to inspire you to boost your intake, check out www.fruitsandveggies.org.

How many different colored veggies and fruits are you getting each day?

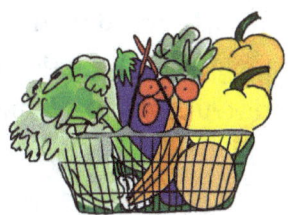

Notes:

> **9** **For a phytonutrient payload, eat more salads.**

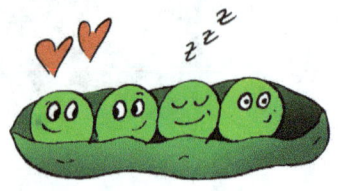

Hap-PEA-ness is being together
—Anonymous

Salads are great, when done right. Here's how to build one that keeps the nutrients high and the calories low, so you can enjoy every bite.

1. Fill your plate with leafy greens. Spinach, romaine lettuce and other leafy greens are great salad starters. (25 calories per 2 cups)

2. Load up on non-starchy veggies. Artichokes, broccoli, cucumbers and other non-starchy veggies are low-calorie, phytonutrient-packed choices. (25 calories per cup)

3. Add starchy veggies in moderation. Beans, corn, lentils, peas and other starchy veggies are rich in complex carbs, but higher in calories. (80 calories per ½ cup)

4. Go easy on extras that add up fast. For a 2-tablespoon serving, typical calories are: dressing (120 calories), nuts and seeds (90 calories), raisins (60 calories), avocado (45 calories) and olives (45 calories).

■ ■ ■

To Do: At least once this week, eat a better salad.

Navigating the salad bar

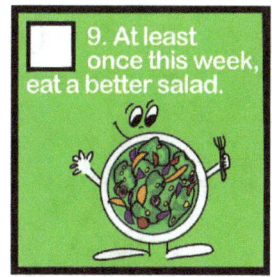

When you're filling your plate at a salad bar, here are five tips to keep in mind so you can make a better salad every time:

- **Get a good perspective.** Before adding anything to your plate, look at what's ahead in line so you can choose what you really want.
- **Build a strong foundation.** Start with green leafy veggies, then add other veggies.
- **Paint a colorful rainbow.** Choose veggies and fruits in a wide range of colors because each color provides different health-promoting properties.
- **Add a protein boost.** For each ounce (about the size of a ping-pong ball) of chicken, tuna, cheese or other protein-rich food, you'll add 7 grams of protein to your salad (45 to 100 calories per ounce.)
- **Take your time.** Smaller bites and more time chewing will help you better digest your food.

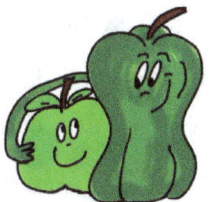

Notes:
_____
_____
_____

> **10** **To detoxify and fortify your health, eat more cruciferous veggies.**

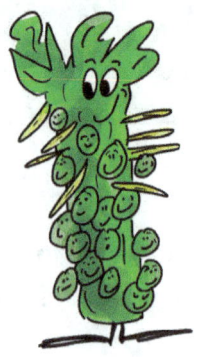

Your liver is a 24/7 detoxifying marvel, and eating more vegetables in the cruciferous family helps it do its job. Think veggies like arugula, bok choy, broccoli, Brussels sprouts, cabbage, cauliflower, collard greens, kale and turnips.

The mind that opens to a new idea never returns to its original size.
— Albert Einstein

Here's how they work. These veggies are a natural source of isothiocyanates, indoles and other phytonutrients with tongue-twister names. These plant compounds help rev up your liver's production of enzymes that trap and remove toxins from your body.

If you need inspiration to eat more of these liver protectors, channel your inner chef. Experiment with infused oils and vinegars, unfamiliar spices and herbs and uncommon forms of veggies like Brussels sprouts on the stalk.

In other words, tap into your natural curiosity to find delicious ways to eat more cruciferous veggies.

Your liver will thank you.

■ ■ ■

To Do: Eat one cruciferous vegetable at least three times this week.

Tap, tap, tap

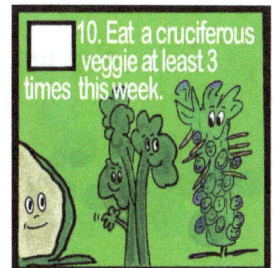

Tap into your natural curiosity to add new cruciferous vegetables to your daily plate. Purple cauliflower, anyone? Then, channel your inner chef to make your dishes as delicious as possible. Here are three ways to get started:

1 **Try infused oils and vinegars.** From olive oil infused with garlic to balsamic vinegar infused with black cherry and beyond, there's no shortage of fun options to try.

2 **Grow your own herbs.** You'll have fresh options to use in your recipes, and fresh herbs tend to be more flavorful than dried varieties. Basil, oregano, thyme, rosemary, parsley, dill and mint are great choices for an herb garden.

3 **Cook a chef-inspired recipe.** Sweet or savory, these recipes use food science to elevate the flavor profile, making them extra delicious.

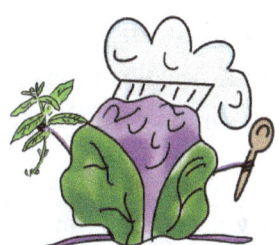

Notes: _____
_____
_____

> **11** **To brighten up a meal, add a colorful grain.**

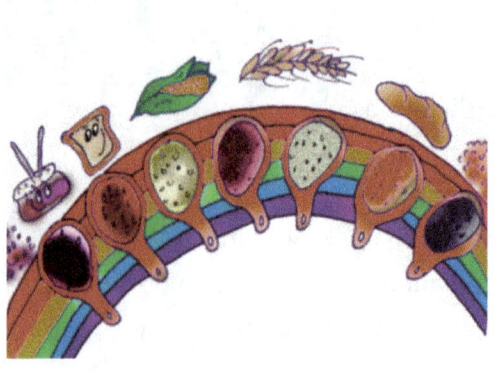

Adding a colorful grain to a meal is a fun way to feed your body the nutrients it needs.

Think essential vitamins and minerals, hunger-curbing fiber and protective phytonutrients.

For a healthy life, eat a colorful diet; for a healthy soul, live a colorful life.
—David J. Greene

For inspiration, check out the bulk food section in your local grocery or health food store. Here, you're sure to find plenty of colorful grains like Himalayan red rice, Chinese black rice or purple Thai rice, just to name a few.

With savory, nutty, fruity and flowery flavors, you might say these colorful grains are a "gRAINBOW" of deliciousness that can take the flavor of just about any dish to a new level.

In other words, colorful grains are good tasting and good for you. What's not to love?

■ ■ ■

To Do: Eat a new colorful grain this week.

Stretch your gRAINBOW

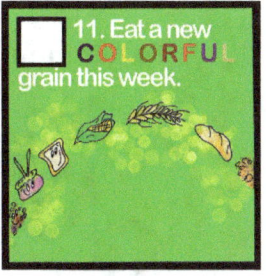

Colorful grains are a nutrient-rich way to add a little pizzazz to your plate. Here's how to get started:

1 **Get creative in the kitchen.** Check out the bulk food bins at your local grocery or health food store. Choose a few grains you haven't tried. Cook them up, and add nuts, dried fruit, seeds, spices and herbs to make your own delicious concoctions.

2 **Be adventurous.** Challenge yourself this week and try one or two new colorful grains. Who knows, you may find one that you really, really like.

3 **Move beyond popcorn.** No doubt, you've snacked on popcorn while doing homework. Why not mix it up with popped sorghum or popped millet?

For more ideas, see **Stretch Your gRAINBOW** on page 102.

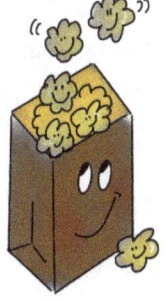

Notes: _____
_____
_____

12   To get more from life, take time to taste.

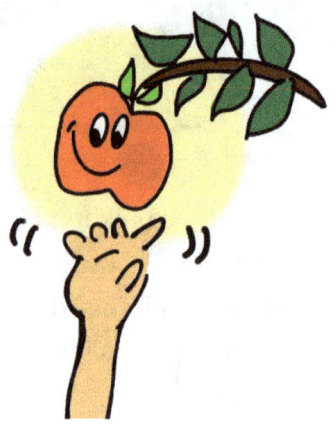

Realize deeply that the present moment is all you have. Make the NOW the primary focus of your life.
—Eckhart Tolle

Have you ever found yourself eating while studying at your desk and reaching for yet another bite only to find you've already scarfed everything down? If so, you're not alone. It's more common than you may think.

Yet, the simple act of paying attention to what you are eating delivers big rewards.

In one study with healthy young adults,[10] researchers found that those who ate a meal slowly (26 minutes) reported more enjoyment and satisfaction compared to those who ate a meal more quickly (6 minutes).

Plus, the slow eaters were less inclined to want to snack a few hours later. All good reasons to slow down and savor the flavor at every meal.

■ ■ ■

To Do: Every day this week, take time to really taste your food.

How to embrace slow eating

Make a deal with yourself. At your next meal, slow down and really taste what you are eating. Is your dish savory? Sweet? Salty? Really taste it and notice how you feel.

Don't forget to take in all the aromas, too. After all, your sense of smell plays a large role in your ability to enjoy food. (Remember how bland your food tasted the last time you had a stuffy nose?)

And, be sure to take part in family meals whenever possible. Why? According to one study,[11] family meals are linked to a whole host of benefits for teens including eating a nutrient-dense diet, feeling better about themselves and more likely to pass on risk-taking behaviors. Plus, the teens who joined in on family meals were just plain happier.

It's a great recipe to be a better you.

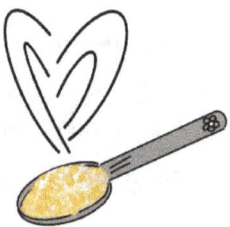

Notes: _____
_____
_____

> **13** To encourage a friend, send inspiring text messages.

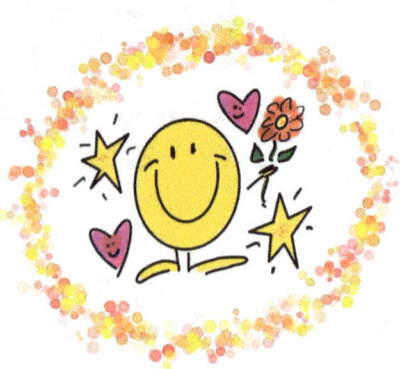

Let us always meet each other with smile, for the smile is the beginning of love.
—Mother Teresa

Your text messages have the power to inspire a friend on their journey to a healthier lifestyle. According to one study,[12] here's what motivates (and what doesn't):

Do text practical tips. Think lunch ideas, success stories about other teens, and positive tips tailored to your friend's individual challenges.

Do text encouraging messages. Think virtual cheerleader, and don't skimp on emoticons and exclamation points. After all, progress toward any healthy goal is nothing short of "Spectacular ☺ !!!"

Don't text about unhealthy foods or behaviors to avoid. Seriously. You may think telling a friend to eat an apple instead of ice cream is helpful, but it's more likely to trigger thoughts of, well, eating ice cream.

In other words, send positive, practical tips. And, don't be shy about congratulating progress along the way.

■ ■ ■

To Do: Every day, help someone be better.

Text messages that inspire others

Here's how you can text positive and practical messages that are sure to inspire a friend to make healthy choices:

1 **Share meal or recipe ideas.** Text a specific tip for a healthy option or substitution. For example, freeze grapes for a refreshing snack, steam carrots with rosemary for a savory flavor boost, or add a lemon slice to sparkling water for a refreshing drink.

2 **Share a helpful strategy that worked for another teen.** For example, "Exercise was boring until I started walking at the mall with my friend. It's more fun to walk and window shop."

3 **Share tailored messages.** Share a tip that targets their individual challenges. For example, if a friend is having trouble eating enough veggies and fruits, sharing a tip about how you eat one of your favorites may help.

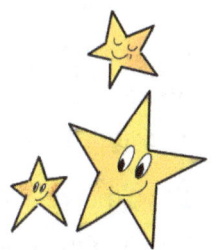

Notes: _____
_____
_____

14   For better heart health, volunteer to help others.

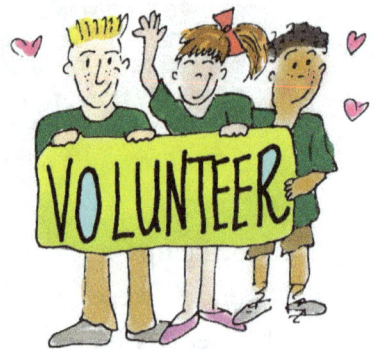

The best way to find yourself is to lose yourself in the service of others.
         —Mahatma Gandhi

If you're among the many teens who volunteer to help others, your good deeds may also be good for your heart health.

One study[13] tells the story. For this study, researchers enrolled more than 100 high school students with similar heart health profiles and randomly assigned them to one of two groups.

One group volunteered with children every week for two months. The other group was placed on a "wait list" for volunteering.

Compared to the wait-list group, the active volunteering group significantly improved three key measures of heart health: blood levels of cholesterol and interleukin-6 (a key marker of inflammation) and body mass index.

Plus, the volunteering teens who were the most empathetic and altruistic or had the biggest improvement in negative mood benefited the most.

■ ■ ■

To Do: Every day, make someone smile.

4 rewards of volunteering

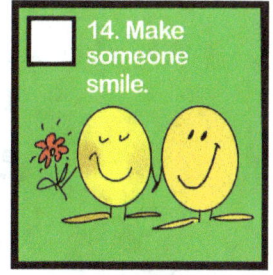

The rewards are great when you volunteer to help others, but only when you take action. Here's some inspiration to get started today:

1 **Focus on what matters to you.** Volunteering is a great way to choose a cause that's meaningful to you.

2 **Learn a new skill.** Volunteering can help you learn a new skill or take on a new challenge (and maybe earn extra credit along the way).

3 **Build on other healthy habits.** Volunteering is a perfect complement to other lifestyle habits needed for a strong heart, habits like eating a healthy diet, getting regular exercise, maintaining a healthy body weight and avoiding smoking cigarettes.

4 **Make a difference in your community.** Volunteering can help you make an impact in your community and boost your sense of pride and satisfaction.

In other words, be present in your interactions, it's a present that goes a long way.

Notes:

> **15** For a happier day, move more.

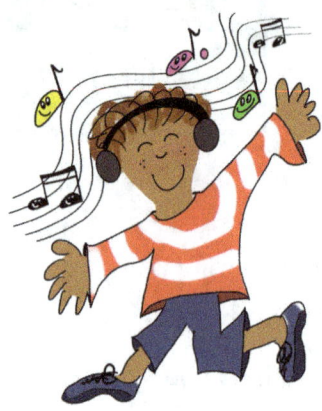

*When in doubt,
turn up the music.*
—Anonymous

You can be happier right now (ok within an hour), you just need to get moving. In general, teens who are more physically active are happier over the long run. But there's also an immediate benefit. In one study,[14] researchers in the Netherlands followed more than 1,480 teens who were given a so-called "wearable lab" that included a wrist fitness tracker and a smartphone. The fitness tracker was used to count steps and track physical activity, minute by minute, for a maximum of 5 days. The smartphone allowed the teens to reply to randomly timed requests to rate how happy they were at that specific moment.

Turns out, the number of steps accumulated in a given hour predicted happiness in the next hour. In fact, adding as few as 1,000 steps to typical daily activity level was enough to shift into happier state of mind for that day (more was better).

For physical health, experts recommend teens get 60 minutes or more of moderate to vigorous activity every day.[15] Adding a few more steps could also mean a happier day.

■ ■ ■

To Do: Every day, move more for a boost of happiness.

4 ways music helps you move more

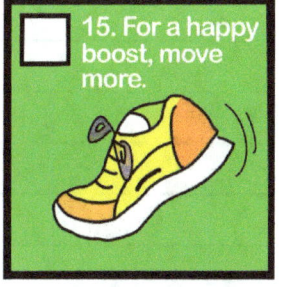

If you need inspiration to get moving to boost your happiness, add a little music to your routine. Here are four research-backed ways music makes it easier for you to stay active every day:[16]

1 **Music makes exercise more enjoyable.** For most teens, this is one of the most important benefits of listening to music while exercising. Why? When exercise is fun, you're more likely to keep at it.

2 **Music helps improve your physical performance.** Tunes with a fast tempo exert a stronger benefit than those with a slow-to-medium tempo. In other words, you move with the tempo of the music.

3 **Music reduces perceived exertion.** Music has the ability to distract you when you feel fatigued or have minor physical discomfort. That is, music makes exercise feel easier.

4 **Music helps improve oxygen consumption.** Being more efficient at using oxygen allows you to delay fatigue and improves your ability to exercise longer.

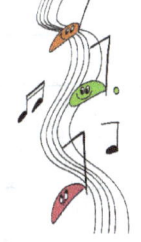

What are your favorite workout songs?

Notes: _____
_____
_____

Notes:

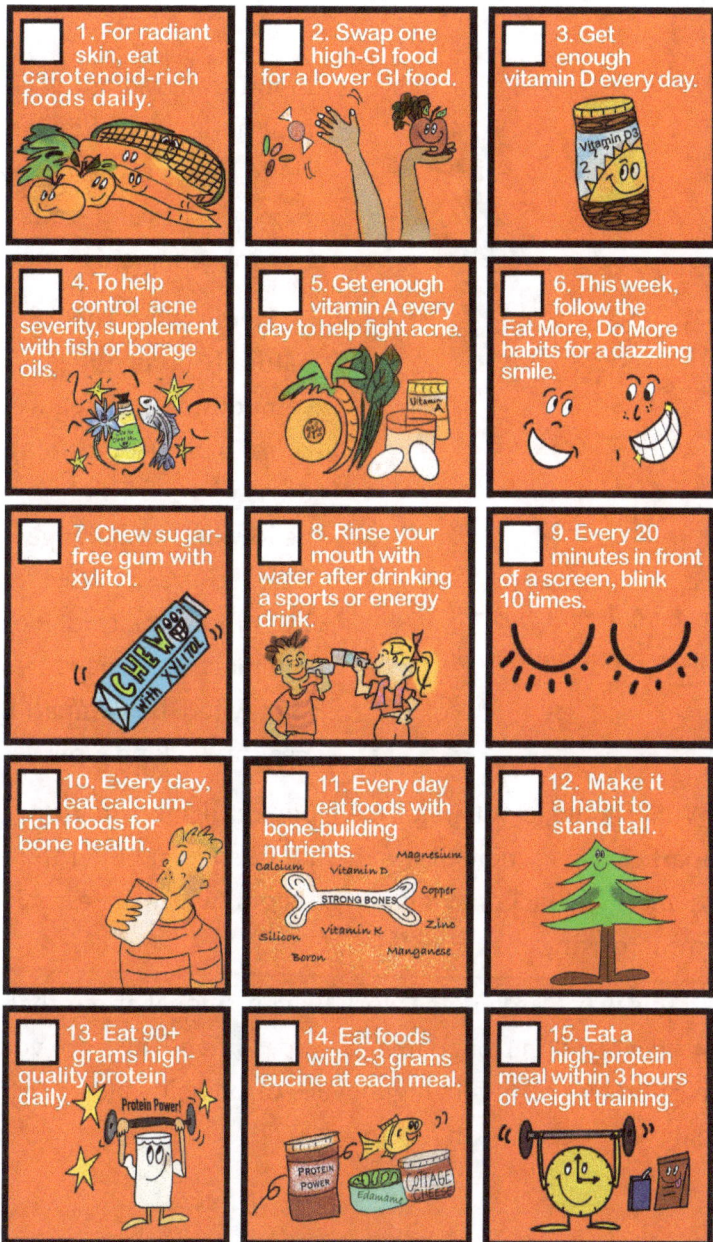

> **1** **To put your best face forward, eat more carotenoid-rich veggies and fruits.**

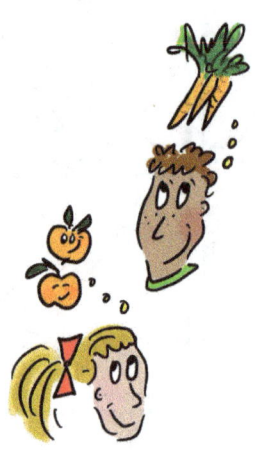

Radiant, healthy looking skin makes every smile brighter.
—*Anonymous*

If you want radiant, healthy-looking skin, it could be as easy as eating more veggies and fruits rich in carotenoids.

Here's why. These naturally occurring compounds impart a warm color to plants, including those you eat. Think yellow, red and orange. Once absorbed in the intestine, some carotenoids can make their way to your skin where they impart a healthy-looking glow.

What's more, carotenoids have powerful antioxidant properties. This action allows them to absorb and filter the high-energy, blue light waves of sunlight, which are especially harmful to skin cells.

In this way, carotenoids work like nutritional armor that protects your skin from damage. And, since all layers of your skin can retain relatively high levels, carotenoids play a critical role in your overall skin health.

■ ■ ■

To Do: Eat carotenoid-rich foods daily (for radiant skin).

Ready, set, glow

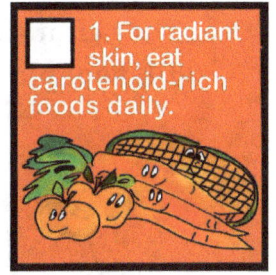

Healthy looking skin isn't all about what you put on your skin, it's also about what you put in your body. To move closer to the radiant skin you want, add three to four servings of carotenoid-rich vegetables and fruits to your daily menu.[17] Here are three simple ways to get started:

1 **Lean towards foods rich in beta-carotene and lycopene.** These are the two carotenoids most likely to give your skin a healthy glow. Apricots, pink grapefruit, carrots and sweet red peppers are a great start. Spinach, kale, broccoli and other greens are good sources too.

2 **Measure for accuracy.** One serving is typically about one cup for raw foods and one-half cup for cooked foods.

3 **Enjoy the reward.** Watch your skin take on a healthy glow in as little as a few weeks.

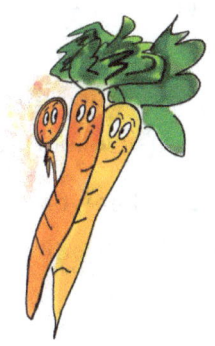

For more carotenoid-rich foods, see **Carotenoid-rich Foods for Healthy Looking Skin** on page 108.

Notes: _____
_____
_____

> **2** **For a clear skin routine that really works, fill your plate with low-GI foods.**

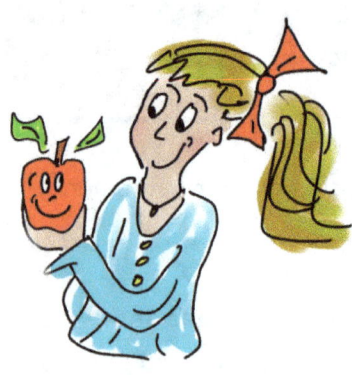

Eat less sugar. You're sweet enough already.
—Anonymous

If you feel like one perfectly placed pimple can shake your confidence, you're not alone. Medical journals are filled with articles about acne and its negative impact on emotional, psychological and social wellbeing.

The good news is more radiant, pimple-free skin can be yours, depending on the foods you choose.

It starts with swapping foods that have a higher glycemic index (GI) with those that have a lower one.

Here's why it matters. When you eat high-GI foods, they tend to cause rapid spikes in your blood sugar. Some scientists say this action directly stimulates the production of hormones responsible for acne.[18]

In other words, choosing low-GI foods more often could be your secret weapon in the fight against acne.

■ ■ ■

To Do: This week, swap one high-GI food for a lower GI food.

How to eat more low-GI foods

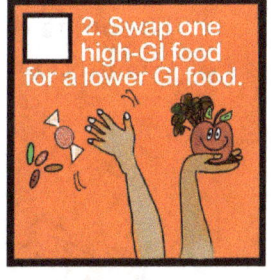

Kickstart your effort to eat more low-GI foods with these simple guidelines:

First, foods that contain little or no carbohydrates are low-GI foods. Think meat, fish, poultry, eggs, avocado and nuts. Non-starchy veggies, for the most part, are also low-GI foods as are dairy products, beans and whole fruits. So, that's easy.

For carbohydrate-rich (starchy) foods, low-GI options tend to be less processed. So, choose whole grain breads and pastas instead of refined, white varieties; brown rice instead of white rice; steel-cut oats or muesli instead of instant oatmeal; boiled white potatoes instead of mashed or instant varieties; and high-fiber, low-sugar breakfast cereals instead of conventional varieties (check the label, and aim for at least 4 grams of fiber and no more than 4 grams of added sugars per serving).

> **Don't overthink this!**
>
> A low-GI food is simply a food that has little effect on raising your blood sugar.

Fruit juices, soda, candy, chips, cookies and other highly processed sugary foods are high-GI foods. So, if you want clear skin, choose these less often.

Notes: _____
_____
_____

> **3**   To soothe dry, itchy winter skin, get enough vitamin D.

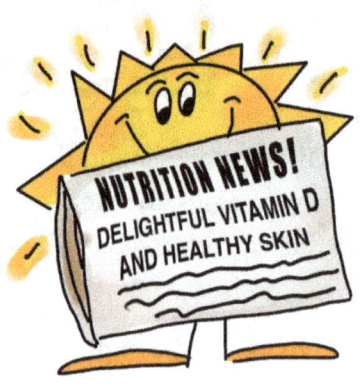

There's plenty of good things about the winter, but seasonal eczema isn't one of them. You'll recognize this common skin condition by itchy, inflamed, red patches of skin that tend to get worse as fall turns to winter.

In the depth of winter, I finally learned that within me there lay an invincible summer.
              —Albert Camus

The good news is winter eczema is no match for the soothing effects of a simple vitamin, say dermatology researchers. Usually, eczema is treated with ultraviolet light therapy, which stimulates vitamin D production in the body. The researchers had a hunch vitamin D supplementation could have a similar effect.

Turns out, it does. In one study[19] with more than 100 kids and teens with winter eczema, those who took a daily vitamin D supplement (1,000 IU per day) for one month reduced the severity of their eczema significantly more than those who took a dummy pill (placebo).

■ ■ ■

To Do: To support healthy winter skin, get enough vitamin D every day.

Sooth winter skin from within

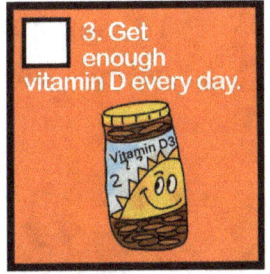

If you suffer from winter-related eczema, combining a daily vitamin D supplement with your regular skin care routine may be just what you need for healthy looking, itch-free skin all winter long.

When choosing a supplement, look for vitamin D3 (cholecalciferol) rather than vitamin D2 (ergocalciferol). Why? Research shows that the D3 form is a more bioavailable form.

You'll find D3 in a wide variety of high-quality multivitamins as well as in single-ingredient supplements.

In addition, it's important to know that, when skin is exposed to the sun, the sunlight stimulates vitamin D production in your body. It's why vitamin D is often called the sunshine vitamin.

So, spend some time in the sun. Aim for about 5 to 30 minutes, two to three times per week from 10 a.m. to 3 p.m. without sunscreen, exposing your face, arms, legs or back to the sun. This is often enough to trigger sufficient vitamin D synthesis to meet your basic vitamin D needs.[20]

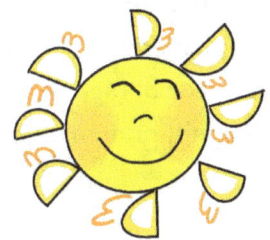

Notes:

> **4** To control acne severity, consume more skin-friendly fats.

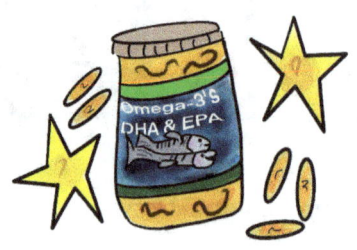

*Happiness is a habit.
So is your skincare.*
—Anonymous

You may be surprised to learn that fish oil and borage oil may help reduce the severity of acne. It's a big reason they're often called skin-friendly fats.

In one study,[21] teens and young adults with mild-to-moderate acne who supplemented with fish oil or borage oil for 10 weeks not only had significantly fewer acne lesions, but also less severe acne than the teens who did not take any supplements.

The researchers point to certain fats in the oils and their ability to reduce inflammation, which is one of the most important disease-causing factors of acne. The fish fats are eicosapentaenoic acid (EPA) and docosahexaenoic acid (DHA). The borage oil fat is gamma-linolenic acid (GLA).

What were the acne-reducing amounts? The fish oil supplement provided 1 gram of EPA and 1 gram of DHA per day. The borage oil supplement provided 0.4 grams (400 milligrams) of GLA per day.

■ ■ ■

To Do: To control acne severity, supplement with fish oil or borage oil.

Fatty acids for clear skin

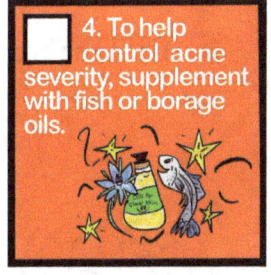
4. To help control acne severity, supplement with fish or borage oils.

Ready to boost your acne-reducing fatty acid intake? Here are three things you need to know:

1 **Eat more fatty fish.** Salmon, haddock, mackerel and other fatty fish can help increase your intake of EPA and DHA. One 4-ounce serving of cooked wild salmon, for example, contains 0.3 grams (300 milligrams) of EPA and 1,200 milligrams of DHA.

2 **Supplement in moderation.** Health experts recommend you consume no more than 5 grams per day of EPA and DHA (combined) from dietary supplements.

3 **Work with your doctor.** If you're considering a fish oil (or borage oil) supplement as part of a treatment program for acne, talk to your doctor first to discuss what's best for your individual needs.

Here's to clear skin!

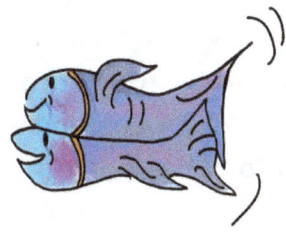

Notes: _____
_____
_____

> **5** To fight acne, turn to the power of vitamin A.

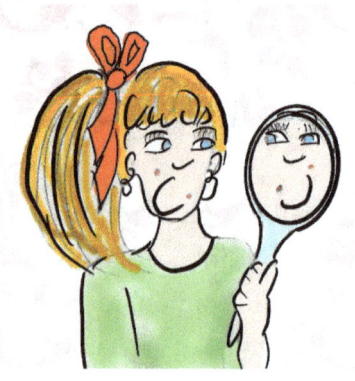

Confidence is the only key. I can't think of any better representation of beauty than someone who is unafraid to be herself.

—Emma Stone

If you're battling acne, you're not alone. In fact, no other skin disorder is as common as *acne vulgaris*. It's a teenage challenge that can have you buying pricey creams, lotions and potions, when nutritional healing may be all you need.

Acne vulgaris is caused by sebum trapped in pores. Sebum is the oily substance that naturally lubricates your skin and hair. But, when sebum clogs a pore, it can promote the growth of bacteria called *Proprionbacterium acnes* or *P. acnes* for short.

UCLA researchers have identified various strains of *P. acnes*, including ones that can shift your immune system into overdrive and cause the inflammation and redness associated with acne.[22] How do you block the pimply actions of *P. acnes*? Consuming an optimal amount of vitamin A can help.[23]

■ ■ ■

To Do: Every day, get enough vitamin A from foods, and supplement to fill any gap.

Zit-zapping effects of vitamin A

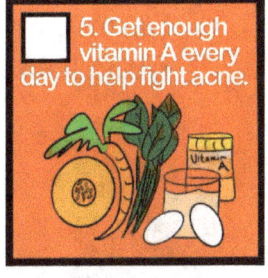

Vitamin A promotes cell turnover, a key action that helps prevent blackheads and whiteheads from forming. Plus, its immune-supporting properties can help control inflammation triggered by acne. Read on for three ways to boost your vitamin A intake for healthy skin:

1 **Fill your plate with colorful veggies and fruits.** Think orange, yellow and green vegetables and fruits like cantaloupe, carrots, kale, spinach and sweet potatoes. These foods contain beta-carotene and other carotenoids that the body can convert into vitamin A (retinol).

2 **Add animal-based foods in moderation.** Foods such as beef and chicken liver, fish, eggs and dairy products are good sources of pre-formed vitamin A in the retinol form.

3 **Take a complete multivitamin with vitamin A.** Look for a supplement that provides up to 100% of the Daily Value for vitamin A per daily serving (from either retinol, beta-carotene or a combination of both).

Notes:

6   To smile bright, fine-tune your food choices and eating habits.

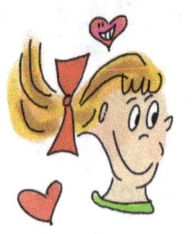 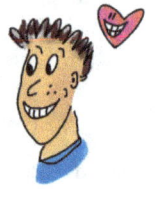

A smile is a curve that sets everything straight.
       —Phyllis Diller

It's amazing how flashing a smile with strong, healthy teeth can deliver a boost in confidence that can leave you feeling like a million dollars.

The good news is you can help prevent cavities from robbing you of your right to feel great by fine-tuning your food choices and eating habits.

In fact, nutritionists agree that you can protect your dazzling smile with two simple dietary habits. First, eat more foods that are associated with fewer cavities. Second, eat in a way associated with fewer cavities.[24]

Think of it as a one-two punch that helps fight dental decay that can keep you from looking good and feeling great. And, it's easier than you may think.

Plus, it's a perfect complement to daily brushing, flossing and regular dental checkups.

■ ■ ■

To Do: This week, follow the Eat More, Do More habits for a dazzling smile.

Eat More, Do More smile habits

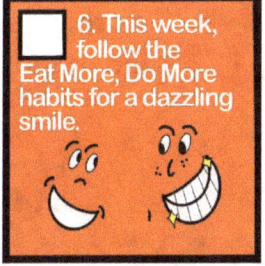

6. This week, follow the Eat More, Do More habits for a dazzling smile.

Do what matters to protect your pearly whites, starting with the Eat More, Do More habits below.

Eat More

- Fresh veggies and fruits
- High-quality protein foods, such as meats, eggs, cheese, fish, beans and legumes
- Whole-grain, low-sugar breads and cereals

Do More

- Space frequency of food and beverage intake at least 2 hours apart.
- Select fresh, whole, unprocessed food to stimulate protective saliva production.
- Avoid frequent and prolonged intakes of sugary foods or sticky foods that cling to teeth (without being accompanied by non-sticky foods).
- Avoid sipping sugar-sweetened beverages for prolonged periods.

Notes: _____
_____
_____

> **7** **To protect your dazzling smile, pick the right kind of gum.**

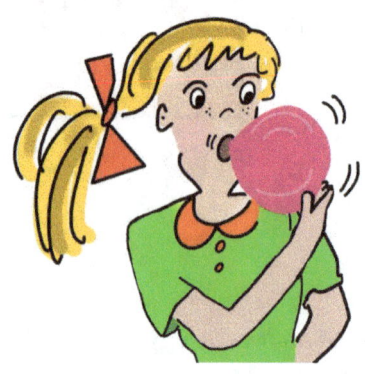

Flattery is like chewing gum. Enjoy it, but don't swallow it.
—*Hank Ketchum*

Some chewing gums can wreak havoc on your teeth, while others actually protect your teeth.

If you want to keep your smile bright and your mouth healthy, you'll want to spot the difference.

The Good "Ol" Ones. Chewing gums that contain sugar alcohols reduce plaque and mouth bacteria. This could mean fewer cavities and a brighter smile. Look for the "ol" at the end of the ingredient names. These include xylit<u>ol</u>, sorbit<u>ol</u> and mannit<u>ol</u>. Of the three, xylitol has the greatest promise for cavity prevention.

The Bad "Ose" Ones. Chewing gums containing sugars increase tooth decay. Look for the "ose" at the end of ingredient names. These include sucr<u>ose</u>, dextr<u>ose</u> and high fruct<u>ose</u> corn syrup. You'll want to avoid these sticky sugar bombs so you can keep your smile bright.

■ ■ ■

To Do: For a brighter smile, chew sugar-free gum with xylitol after meals.

Chew on this

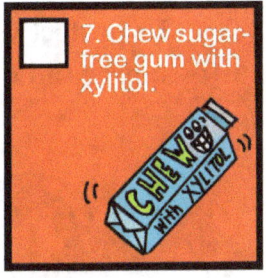

7. Chew sugar-free gum with xylitol.

Chewing a sugar-free, xylitol-containing gum can help protect your teeth, but only when done right. Here's how:

1 **Chew enough.** Make sure xylitol is listed as the first ingredient. If it's listed further down the ingredient list or with another sweetener like sorbitol, the gum is unlikely to deliver enough protective xylitol.

2 **Chew at the right time.** Xylitol gum protects against tooth decay when chewed three to five times per day, after meals, for a total daily intake of at least 5 grams of xylitol per day.[25] If you chew gum with about 2 grams after each meal, you'll hit this target. But don't overdo it, too much xylitol may cause loose stools.

3 **Chew long enough.** Chew a xylitol-containing gum for about 5 minutes after each meal. This helps release enough xylitol into your saliva to fully deliver its toothy benefits.

Notes:

8. To protect your pearly whites, lighten up on sports and energy drinks.

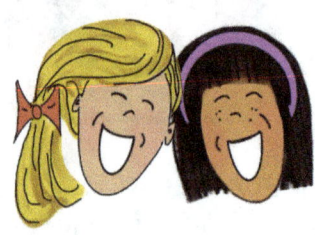

Make a smile your signature accessory.
— Anonymous

If you drink sports and energy drinks, you're not alone. Up to 50% of teens drink energy beverages and over 60% drink at least one sports drink daily.[26] That's a lot of gulping.

The trouble is, along with sugar, these drinks typically contain citric acid. This corrosive combo is like soda on steroids, eating away at your tooth enamel.

One study[26] found exposing teeth to these drinks caused tooth enamel to significantly deteriorate. The researchers looked at nine popular energy drinks and 13 sports drinks. To each drink, they submerged dental enamel for 15 minutes. Next, they transferred the enamel into artificial saliva where it sat for two hours. This procedure occurred five times each day for a total of five days. The result: Both types of drinks were bad news for teeth, but energy drinks were doubly so.

To protect your teeth, your best strategy is to avoid sugary, acidic sports and energy drinks. But, if you really want one, rinsing your mouth with water afterwards can help reduce their dental damage.

■ ■ ■

To Do: Rinse your mouth with water after drinking a sports or energy drink.

3 simple ways to protect your teeth

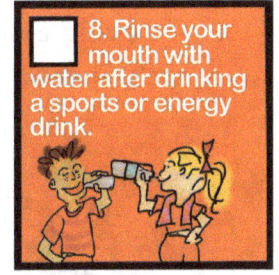

Acidic, sugary sports and energy drinks can erode tooth enamel, promote tooth decay and rob you of your smile. Here are three ways to fight back:

1 **Drink water instead.** Sports drinks can help replenish electrolytes that you lose in sweat during long, grueling activities, but, if you're chugging these drinks while just hanging out, you would be better off switching to water.

2 **Immediately rinse or chew gum.** Rinse out your mouth with water or chew sugarless gum right after you drink. Both actions help increase saliva flow, which helps restore the pH of your mouth to a less acidic, more normal state.

3 **Wait to brush your teeth.** Brushing your teeth can actually spread the acidity to other teeth and increase damage. Better to wait about one hour after you drink to brush.

Notes:

9 — To avoid eye strain, fill your plate with lutein-rich foods and take blinking breaks.

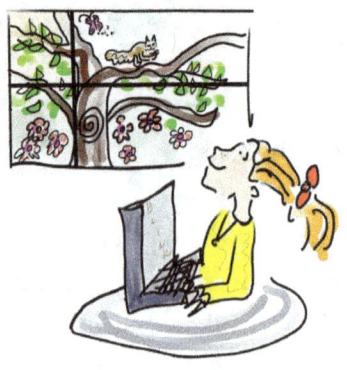

There is no danger of developing eyestrain from looking at the bright side of things.
—Joyce Meyer

If you're like many teens, you're spending more time staring into digital screens. A lot more. Yet, too much screen time can cause eye strain.

You know the feeling: sore, tired, itchy eyes that are either too dry or too watery and often trigger a headache.

Enter lutein, a yellow plant pigment and powerful antioxidant. It's why foods like corn and egg yolks are yellow, but the highest amounts are found in green vegetables like spinach and kale. (It's hiding under the green of chlorophyll.)

Once consumed, lutein travels to the macula, the area of the eye responsible for sharp vision, where it absorbs harmful high-energy blue light (the same light emitted by typical video display screens). Think of it as a nutritional shield for your eyes. Add regular blinking breaks, and you just may banish tired, sore eyes for good.

■ ■ ■

To Do: Every 20 minutes in front of a screen, blink 10 times to soothe and rewet your eyes.

Blinking basics to avoid eye strain

9. Every 20 minutes in front of a screen, blink 10 times.

We tend to blink less frequently when gazing into a digital screen, which can lead to dry, irritated eyes. You can help avoid this nuisance by taking regular blinking breaks. Here's how:

1 **Use the 20-20-20 Rule.** Look away from your screen for 20 seconds and focus your gaze on something at least 20 feet in the distance. Do this every 20 minutes you're behind a screen. (If you find it hard to remember, set a timer as a reminder to take a break.)

2 **Keep your screen at arm's length.** For better eye comfort, keep any screen (computer, laptop, tablet, phone) at least 18 to 24 inches from your eyes (about arm's length).

3 **Rewet your eyes, naturally.** Take a blinking break to help rewet your eyes and promote eye comfort. Blink 10 times (very slowly) every 20 minutes.

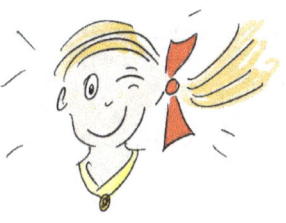

Notes: _____
_____
_____

10 To unleash your growth potential, get enough calcium.

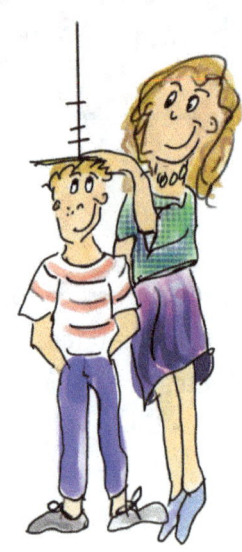

Don't go through life, grow through life.
—Eric Butterworth

You have the ability to realize your full height naturally, but only if you start now. Why? By your 18th birthday, virtually all your adult skeleton is formed.

Bone is a dynamic tissue, and it's in a constant state of turnover at every stage of life. But, during the teen years, bone formation shifts into overdrive.

For this reason, your body needs all the bone-building nutrients it can get right now if it's to build the strong, sturdy bones you need to reach your full growth potential.

One key nutrient is calcium. Nutrition experts recommend teens consume 1,300 milligrams every day. (That's 100% of the Daily Value.) The good news is you'll find calcium listed on food and supplement labels, so you have a ready resource to make sure you're consuming enough.

Start now, and your future self will thank you.

■ ■ ■

To Do: Every day, eat calcium-rich foods for bone health, and supplement to fill any gap.

3 ways to boost your calcium intake

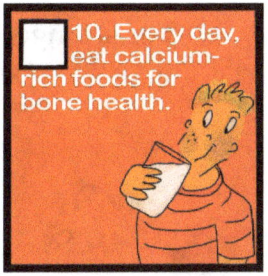

1 **Eat more calcium-rich foods.** Dairy products are typically rich in calcium. For example, one cup of milk provides about 300 milligrams of calcium (23% of the Daily Value), while one cup of yogurt provides about 400 milligrams (31% of the Daily Value). Other good food sources include kale, spinach, broccoli and other dark green, leafy vegetables as well as canned fish, almonds and beans.

2 **Read food labels.** When a packaged food contains 2% or more of the Daily Value for calcium, you'll find it listed in the label's Nutrition Facts box. It's a handy way to check how much calcium is in any packaged food you eat.

3 **Take a multi.** A daily multivitamin helps fill a nutrient gap between what's on your daily plate and what your body needs to fully nourish your bone health. Many quality multis provide about 10% or more of the Daily Value for calcium.

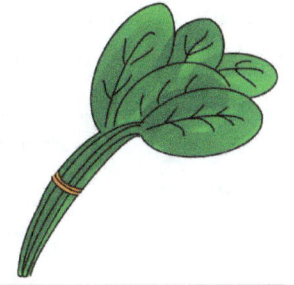

Notes:
_____
_____
_____

11 For stronger bones, know all the nutrients that matter.

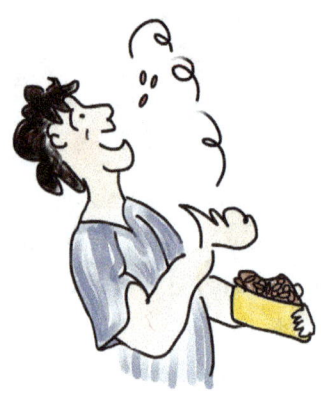

To thrive in life, you need three bones: A wish bone. A backbone. And a funny bone.

—Reba McEntire

Your teenage body is a 24/7 bone-building machine, primed to drink in all the nutrients you can send its way.

Enjoy a salmon filet, and your body grabs vitamin D to boost calcium absorption and zinc to support the structural integrity of your bones. Serve up a spinach salad, and your body extracts vitamin K to make key bone-forming proteins. Munch on nuts, and your body seizes magnesium, copper and manganese, all essential minerals that help activate biochemical pathways needed to build strong bones.

While calcium reigns supreme as the king of teenage bone-building nutrients, it's unable to do its job without the help of other nutrients. In other words, if you want to achieve peak bone mass during your teen years, now is the time to fill your plate with a wide variety of foods with bone-building nutrients.

■ ■ ■

To Do: Eat foods with bone-building nutrients daily, and supplement to fill any gaps.

Bone nutrients beyond calcium

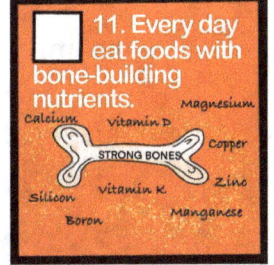

You may not be surprised to know that you need calcium to build strong bones. What may surprise you is your body needs a whole slew of other nutrients to fully activate all the biochemical pathways critical for building and maintaining strong bones.

The good news is you'll find one or more bone-building nutrient in familiar foods such as milk and other dairy products, green veggies, nuts and seeds, whole grains and legumes. If you're seeing a theme here (eat a variety of foods), you're right.

Here's the list of key vitamins and minerals you need to build strong bones:

- Calcium
- Vitamin D
- Vitamin K
- Magnesium
- Copper
- Manganese
- Zinc
- Boron
- Silicon

To learn more about these nutrients, how they work to build strong bones and what foods are good sources, see **Key Bone-building Nutrients** on page 110.

Notes: _____
_____
_____

> **12** To instantly look better, stand tall.

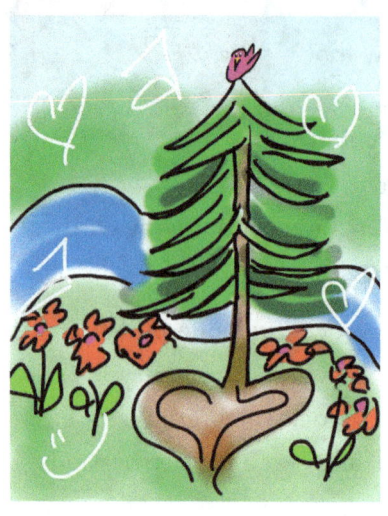

Don't let anyone fool you. It takes effort to shape the diet and lifestyle habits you need to feel good (and look good).

It's why you should celebrate even small changes like drinking water instead of soda, snacking on popcorn instead of chips, or eating fresh strawberries instead of ice cream for dessert.

Advice from a Tree
Stand tall and proud.
Go out on a limb.
Remember your roots.
Drink plenty of water.
Be content with your natural beauty.
Enjoy the view.
—Ilan Shamir

Why? Small changes like these add up to the ultimate prize of a healthier you. But there's no reason you can't instantly look better. How? Stand up straight.

Go ahead, give it a try. Pull your shoulders back and hold your head high. Standing up straight, instead of slouching, has the same effect as gaining up to one inch. Plus, it does double duty as a type of power pose that could help boost your confidence in social settings.[27]

■ ■ ■

To Do: Make it a habit to stand tall.

3 steps to look better

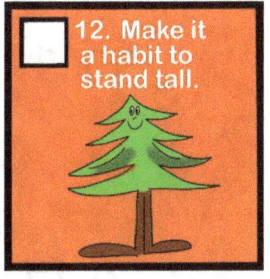

You can take a lesson from classically trained dancers and their techniques for perfect posture. The good news is you don't need years of dance classes to master these moves. Instead, you only need to follow three simple steps:

1 **Pull your shoulders back.** When standing around, imagine you have a straight rod holding you up from head to toe.

2 **Avoid "sitting on a hip."** If you stand slouched to one side (what dancers call "sitting on a hip"), you change your center of gravity and increase pressure on the supporting hip. Instead, stand with your weight equally distributed between both legs, and you'll look taller and leaner.

3 **Hold your head high.** Save the texting for another time. Hold your head up and look forward as you stand and walk.

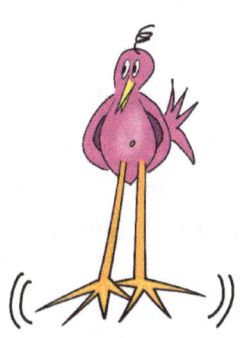

Notes:

13   For muscle building, eat enough protein.

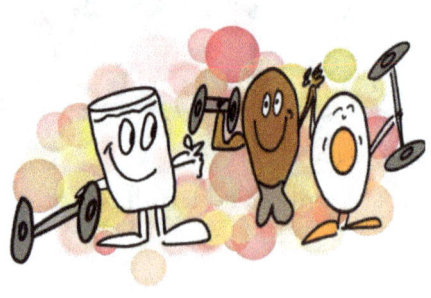

When life gives you lemons, ask for something higher in protein.
                        —*Anonymous*

Whether your goal is to build muscle mass or improve muscle tone, you want to see results fast. Combining a healthy protein-rich diet with your weight training program can help.

The amount of protein you eat every day—in fact, the amount you eat at every meal—affects how your muscles respond to weight training.

Here's a rule of thumb: Consume at least 90 grams of high-quality protein each day, and divide it evenly among your three main meals. This strategy helps maximize muscle protein synthesis and leads to a muscle-building response within 24 hours.

Protein is found in animal foods like meat, fish, poultry and eggs and in some plant foods like beans, grains and vegetables. Other food groups like fruits or fats like butter and oils lack protein.

■ ■ ■

To Do: Eat at least 90 grams of high-quality protein daily (for muscle building and toning).

Where's the protein?

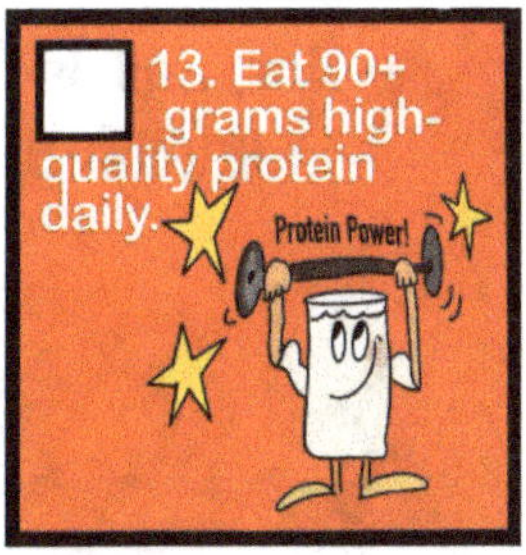

13. Eat 90+ grams high-quality protein daily. Protein Power!

Here's a sample menu with at least 30 grams of protein per meal:

Breakfast
Scrambled eggs (2 medium eggs,*
 1 ounce cheese,* salsa)
Banana toast (1 slice whole grain toast,* 1 tablespoon almond
 butter,* ½ medium banana)
1 cup low-fat milk*

Lunch
Turkey pita pocket (1 whole wheat pita,* 3 ounces turkey,*
 1 ounce cheddar cheese,* lettuce, tomato, mustard)
Sparkling water
1 apple

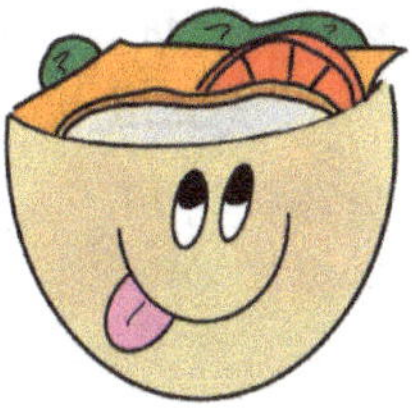

Dinner
1 cup bean soup*
2 cups mixed green salad*
1 sweet potato*
½ cup steamed broccoli*
1 whole grain roll* with 1 teaspoon butter
1 cup low-fat milk*
¾ cup blueberry sorbet

*Protein source

For more protein-rich foods, see **Where's the Protein?** on page 112.

Notes: _____
_____
_____

> **14** **For muscle building, choose protein foods rich in leucine.**

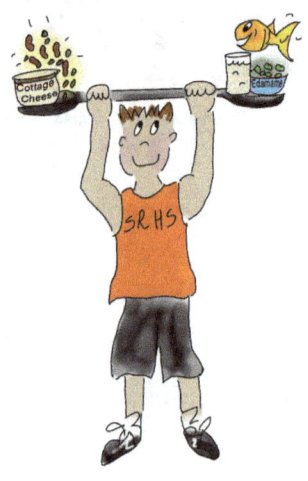

Whether you think you can, or think you can't, you're right.

—Henry Ford

Eating enough protein is a great start to build and tone muscles. But, if you want to take your efforts to the next level, you'll also want to make sure the protein foods you choose are rich in one amino acid: leucine.

Some fitness experts call leucine a "trigger" for muscle synthesis. Why? Unlike other amino acids, leucine appears to have a muscle-building effect. So, you'll want your main meals to provide at least 30 grams of protein, but you'll also want them to deliver about 2 to 3 grams of leucine.[28]

Simplify things by choosing high-quality protein foods like lean chicken, beef or pork, or low-fat dairy products. These foods are rich in both protein and leucine. Protein-rich plant foods such as soybeans also deliver an impressive amount of leucine without a lot of extra calories.

■ ■ ■

To Do: Eat protein foods with 2 to 3 grams of leucine per meal (for muscle building and toning).

3 ways to boost your leucine intake

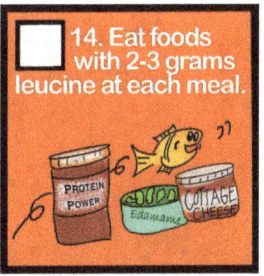

If you want to get enough leucine at each meal, adding a quality protein powder can help. Here's what to look for:

1 **Read labels.** Choose a product that lists its amino acid profile on the label. While it's not required, quality brands include it.

2 **Recognize different units of measure.** Some brands of protein powder list leucine (and other amino acids) on the label in grams; others use milligrams. (One gram equals 1,000 milligrams.) So, one pea protein powder may use 1.7 grams of leucine per scoop on its label, while another uses 1,700 milligrams to describe the same amount.

3 **Be creative.** Go beyond the typical protein shake to sprinkle protein powder into your meals. Mix a scoop into cereal, yogurt, soup or other foods.

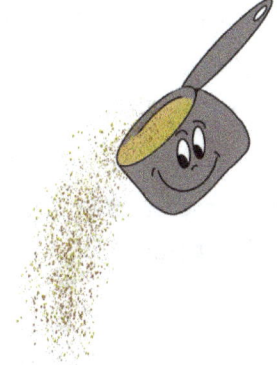

For food sources of leucine, see **Where's the Leucine?** on page 114.

Notes:

> **15** **For muscle building, eat protein foods at the right time.**

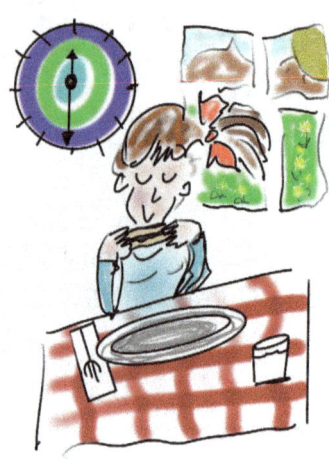

Life is about timing.
—Carl Lewis

In addition to eating enough protein and muscle-building leucine (see previous tips), you'll want to time your intake relative to your workout schedule. This is the final step to maximize the muscle building and toning benefits of a high-protein diet.

Why? Sports nutrition experts report that consuming 20 to 40 grams of high-quality protein maximizes the rate of muscle protein synthesis for three to four hours following exercise.[29] In other words, the right post-workout meal can make a big difference in your ability to build and tone your muscles, whether your goal is to excel in sports or simply look and feel great.

The bottom line: Maximize the muscle benefits of your weight training efforts by eating a high-protein diet the 1-2-3 way: Amount, Type and Timing.

■ ■ ■

To Do: Eat a high-protein meal within 3 hours of weight training (for muscle building and toning).

Post-exercise recovery

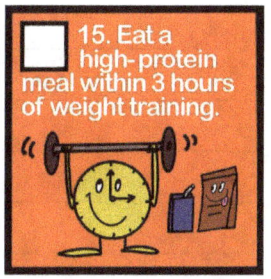

Without enough rest between weight-training sessions, you're more likely to tear down muscle and undo all your hard work. Here's how to recover like a pro:

1 **Get enough rest.** Resist the urge to overdo it in the gym. Wait a day between sessions or, at the very least, work different sets of muscles on consecutive days.

2 **Eat before a workout.** If you expect your next protein-rich meal to be more than 3 hours after a workout, consider eating before you hit the weight room. Not only will this fuel your workout, it will help optimize muscle protein synthesis.

3 **Keep a food log.** You can easily keep track of your protein and leucine intake by using a simple composition book to log your food intake. It's a great way to make sure you're eating a high-protein diet the 1-2-3 way.

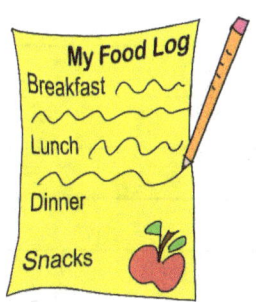

Notes: _____
_____
_____

Notes:

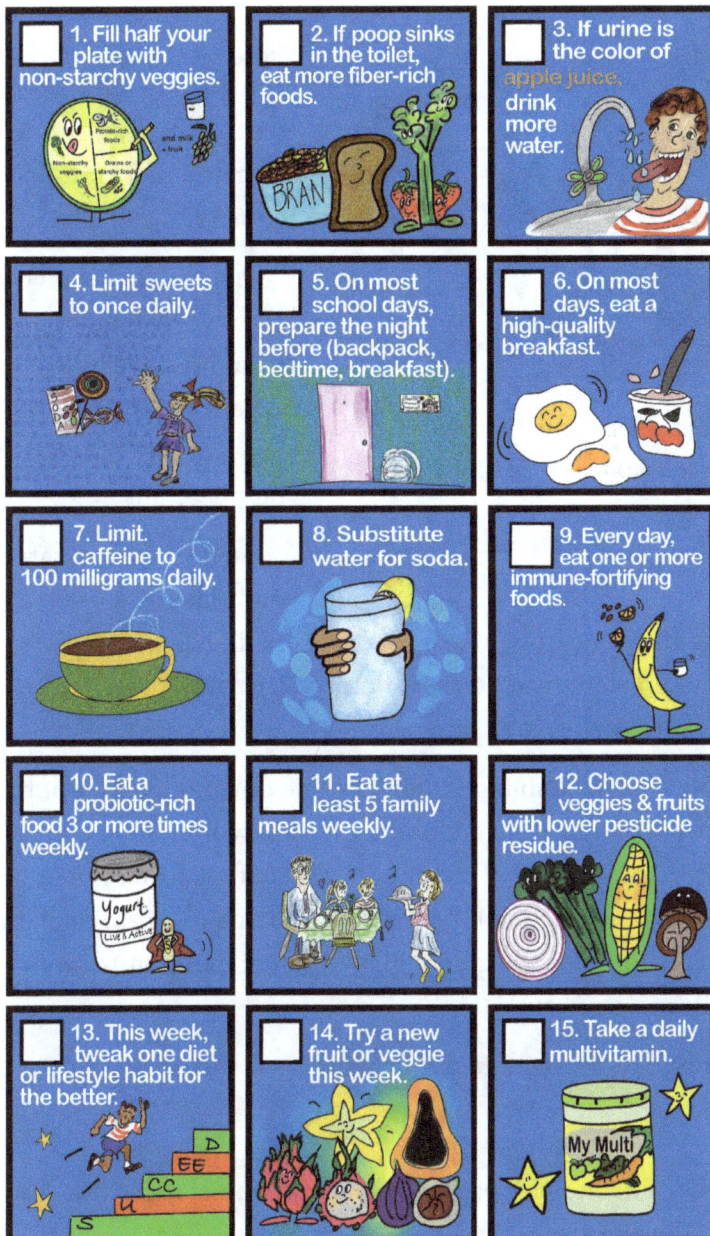

1   To be your best, fill your plate for performance.

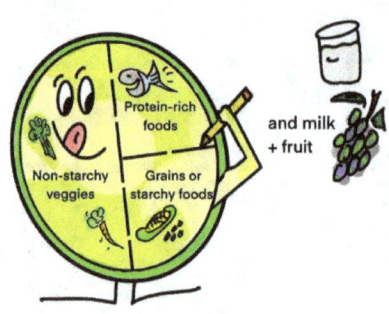

A wise man ought to realize that health is his most valuable possession.

—*Hippocrates*

It's a good bet that you want all the energy you can get to fuel your daily activities.

One way to keep your energy level high throughout the day is to fill your plate the right way. And, it's easier than you may think.

First, take a look at your plate, and draw an imaginary line down the middle. Then, fill half of the plate with non-starchy veggies like broccoli, carrots, cauliflower, tomatoes or zucchini, among others.

Next, draw another imaginary line down the center of the empty half of the plate, dividing it into two sections. Use one section for grains and starchy foods like rice, corn or potatoes. Use the other section for protein-rich foods like fish, chicken, meat or tofu. Finally, add a glass of low-fat or non-fat milk and a piece of fruit.

Preparing to conquer your world is that simple.

■ ■ ■

To Do: Fill one-half of your plate with non-starchy veggies.

Sizing up your food portions

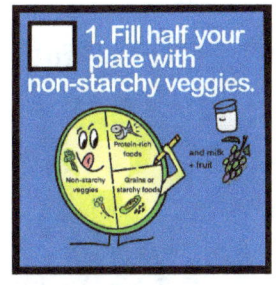

Understanding food portions may seem hard, but you can make it easier simply by using your hand as a guide.

Not only is your hand convenient, it's a surprisingly accurate measuring tool to estimate food portions. Here's the breakdown:

- **Your palm.** A 3-ounce serving of a protein-rich food like meat, fish or chicken is about the same size as the palm of your hand (or a deck of playing cards).

- **Your fist.** A one-cup serving of milk, yogurt or fresh greens is about the same size as your fist.

- **Your cupped hand.** A one-half cup serving of fruit, cooked vegetables or pasta is about the size of your cupped hand (or half a tennis ball).

- **Your thumb.** A one-ounce serving of cheese is about the size of your thumb.

- **Your thumb tip.** A one-teaspoon serving of oil, butter or margarine is about the same size as your thumb tip to the first knuckle.

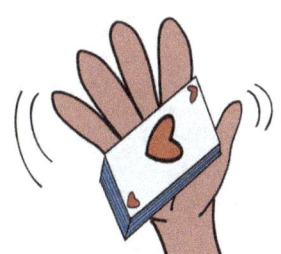

Notes: _____

_____

_____

2   To feel full and satisfied, eat enough fiber.

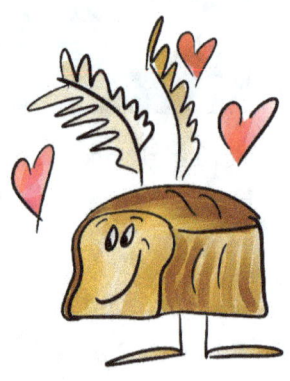

I love you with every fiber of my being.
—Anonymous

If you're like many teens, you probably don't give dietary fiber a second thought. It's understandable. After all, we don't know what we don't know.

Yet, what if you knew that study after study points to the health benefits of fiber. How fiber helps you curb your appetite so you can feel full. How it helps you maintain a strong heart and keep your blood sugar in balance. How fiber helps keep your digestive tract humming along so you can stay regular and prevent constipation.[30] And, how getting enough fiber can even brighten your mood.[31]

It's an impressive body of research, and it all points to one simple rule: For every 1,000 calories you eat, consume 14 grams of fiber.

In practical terms, this means a daily fiber intake of about 26 grams for a teenage girl and about 38 grams for a teenage boy.

■ ■ ■

To Do: Check your poop daily. If it sinks in the toilet, boost your fiber intake.

Turning sinkers into floaters

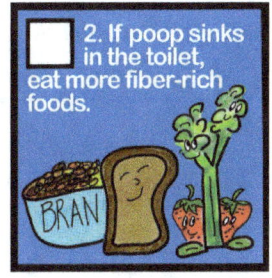

One way to see if you're getting enough fiber is to check your poop. Yes, your poop.

If it floats, that's a good indication that you're getting enough fiber in your diet. On the other hand, if it's a sinker, right to the bottom of the toilet bowl, it's time to boost your fiber intake.

You'll only find fiber in plant foods. It's nowhere to be found in animal foods, not even in the toughest steak. Zip, zero, zilch.

In other words, if you want to boost your fiber intake, you'll need to eat more plant foods. Think vegetables, fruits, dried beans and peas, nuts and seeds, and whole grains.

The good news is, with so much variety, it's easy to choose plant foods that are both delicious and rich in fiber.

A word of caution: Be sure to increase your fiber intake slowly. Too much, too fast can upset your stomach and leave you with digestive upset. For good food sources of fiber, see **Where's the Fiber?** on page 116.

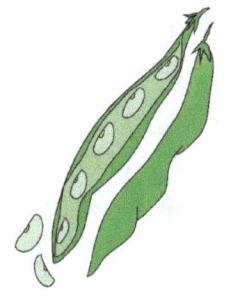

Notes: _____
_____
_____

> **3** **To make sure you're fully hydrated, take a look at your pee.**

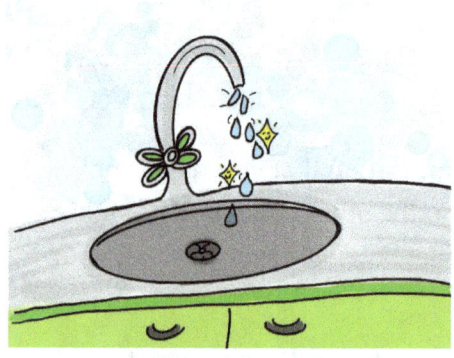

Water is the driving force of all nature.
—Leonardo da Vinci

Did you know that you can live for weeks without food, but only a few days without water? That's how important staying properly hydrated is to your overall wellbeing.

For starters, water is needed to transport nutrients throughout your body, eliminate toxic byproducts, and keep you from overheating by getting rid of excess heat through sweat.

Teenage girls need about 10 to 11 cups of water per day, and teenage boys need about 14 to 15 cups daily.[32] This comes from the water you consume in beverages and drinking water (about 80%) and from the water you get in the foods you eat (about 20%). For active teens, here's a good rule-of-thumb: Weigh yourself before and after vigorous exercise. For every pound you lose, drink an extra 2 to 3 cups of water to replenish and rehydrate.

■ ■ ■

To Do: Look at your urine every day. Drink more water if it's the color of apple juice.

A urine checklist for hydration

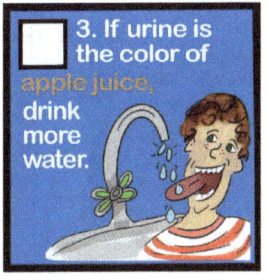

Here are three ways you can use your urine to tell you if you're properly hydrated:

1 **Gauge the color.** Before flushing the toilet, look at your urine. If it's the color of apple juice, you're likely dehydrated and need to drink more. If it's the color of lemonade, you're probably well hydrated.

2 **Take a whiff.** Smelly urine could be a sign that you're dehydrated and need to drink more. Although, some people have stinky urine after eating asparagus. It's a genetic thing. Either they're better able to digest asparagus, or they have a more finely tuned sense of smell. Either way, it's normal, just smelly.

3 **Count to 21.** On average, nearly all mammals take 21 seconds to pee, according to one study.[33] So, if you take less time, you may need to drink more water.

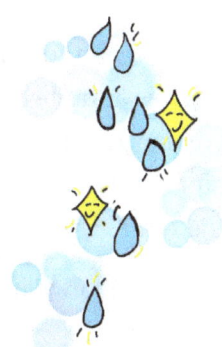

Notes:
_____
_____

4   To control inflammation, say goodbye to added sugars.

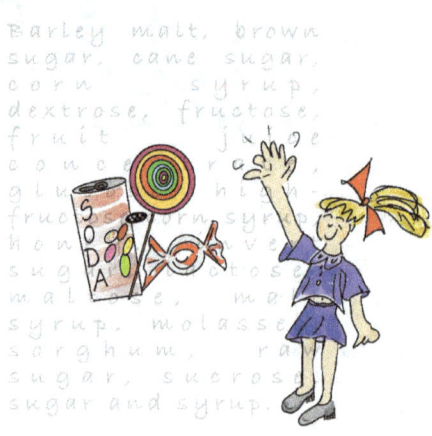

Stressed spelled backwards is Desserts. Coincidence? I think not!
—Anonymous

It may be time to say goodbye to eating too much added sugars. Why? Consuming too many of these empty calories can lead to chronic, low-grade inflammation, compromise your health, and even sour your outlook.[34]

Yet, a typical teen diet packs 17 teaspoons per day.[35] One big culprit is packaged foods and beverages.[36] A 12-ounce can of regular soda, for example, has 10 teaspoons of sugar.

Instead, aim to consume no more than 10% of your daily calories as added sugars.[37] In practical terms, this means no more than 12½ teaspoons (50 grams or 200 calories) of added sugars per day for a 2,000-calorie intake. Of course, the less, the better.

The good news is you can easily spot added sugars in packaged foods with a little label reading savvy, so you can move on to healthier choices faster.

■ ■ ■

To Do: Limit sugary sweets to once daily.

Say so long to added sugars

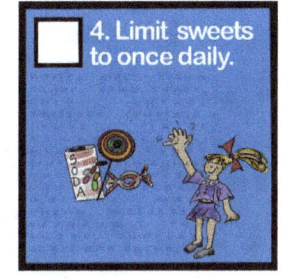

1 **Use a cold turkey approach.**
Go one week without foods high in added sugars. The first few days may be tough. That's no surprise. What may surprise you is, the longer you keep it up, the easier it gets.

2 **Look in the Nutrition Facts box.** Packaged foods are required to list added sugars (in grams) in this part of the label (even if the food has no added sugars). In this way, you can quickly see how much (or how little) added sugars is in the food.

3 **Read the ingredient list.** With a few exceptions, sugar (or another term for sugar) listed among the first three ingredients of a packaged food is a clue the food is likely high in added sugars. For example, honey, barley malt and corn syrup are sugars as is anything that ends in "ose" like fructose (fruit sugar), lactose (milk sugar) and sucrose (table sugar).

> **Seeing is believing**
>
> Scoop 10 teaspoons of sugar into a cup. You're looking at the amount found in 12 ounces of regular soda and 160 calories with little nutritional value (empty calories).

Notes:

5 To be ready for early morning zero periods, prepare the no-brainer way.

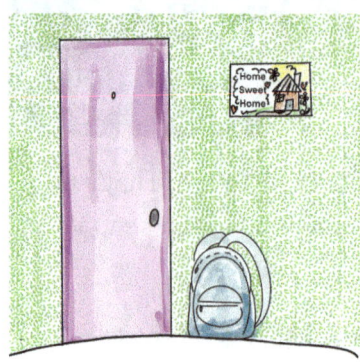

A beautiful day begins with a beautiful mindset.
—*John Geiger*

If you're a ambitious teen, it's a good bet that you have a "zero period" to work on leadership skills, sports training, music classes or another passion.

The trouble is, all zero periods are early morning classes. You need to be up at dawn, out the door and ready to go by 7 a.m.

All that extra classroom time is great. It's even better when you prepare the night before by packing your backpack, having your breakfast plans in order and getting a restful night's sleep.

In this way, you avoid the morning scramble (and the headache that comes with it). Instead, you'll start your school day feeling rested and ready to learn, even during zero period.

■ ■ ■

To Do: On school days, prepare the night before with the three B's: backpack, breakfast and bedtime.

Your zero period, only better

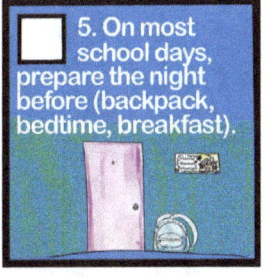

☐ 5. On most school days, prepare the night before (backpack, bedtime, breakfast).

You can get the most out of an early morning zero period when you prepare the night before, starting with the three B's: backpack, breakfast and bedtime.

1 **Backpack.** Pack and place your backpack by the door the night before. Include everything you need for the next day. Everything.

2 **Bedtime.** You need about 9 hours of sleep every night to feel fully rested. Don't be tempted to skimp on it. It's when your brain actively converts new information into long-term memory.

3 **Breakfast.** Squeeze in a healthy breakfast. If you are being driven to school, grab your breakfast and eat it in the car. Think portable foods that don't spill. (For quick breakfast ideas see **Breakfast in Under 5 Minutes** on page 126.)

Notes: _____
_____
_____

6 For benefits that last all day, eat a high-protein breakfast.

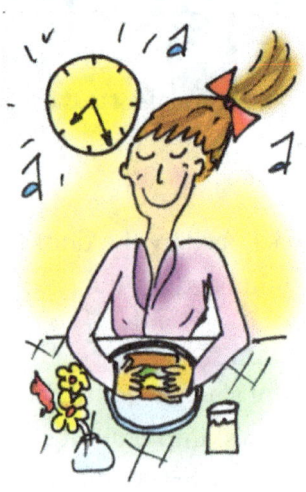

Have a smile for breakfast and you'll be sharing joy for lunch.
—Joe Abercrombie

You may know eating a high-protein breakfast before a morning workout helps you build and tone muscles. This is especially true when you choose high-quality protein foods that are also rich in the amino acid leucine, foods like lean chicken, tofu or low-fat dairy.

What you may not know is a high-protein breakfast delivers other benefits, ones that last all day long.

For example, eating a high-protein breakfast (35 grams of protein) instead of skipping breakfast can help you feel full, eat fewer calories throughout the day (voluntarily) and even avoid gaining excess body fat.[38] A high-protein breakfast can also help you keep your blood sugar on an even keel throughout the day (and avoid mood swings).[39] Plus, a high-quality breakfast (with protein) helps improve morning mental tasks like attention, focus and memory.[40] It all adds up to body (and brain) benefits too good to pass up.

■ ■ ■

To Do: On most days, eat a high-quality breakfast.

Breakfast protein made easy

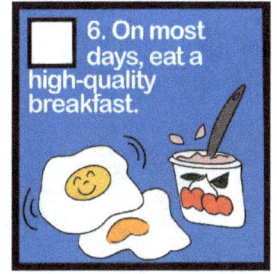

There are plenty of ways you can add more protein to your morning meal like eggs, peanut butter, dried beans, milk, yogurt, cheese, nuts, seeds and more.

Even a high-protein breakfast bar or a smoothie with protein powder can do in a pinch for a grab-and-go breakfast.

And, one of the best ways you can increase your odds of starting your day with a hearty breakfast is to plan the night before.

Here's how: Before you go to bed, give it some thought and make sure you have everything you need at the ready.

In this way, your morning prep time will be faster, giving you more time to enjoy a delicious breakfast to fuel your day.

For protein-rich recipes, see **Power Smoothie Recipes** on page 120. (While these recipes support muscle building and toning, they can do double duty as high-protein breakfast options.)

Notes:

7 To banish caffeine jitters, find your Goldilocks balance.

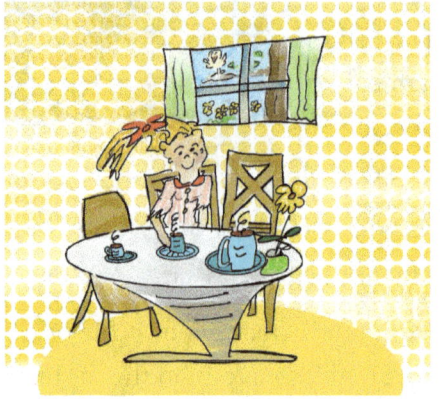

I never drink coffee at lunch. I find it keeps me awake for the afternoon.

— *Ronald Reagan*

Do you find yourself jittery? Anxious? Does your heart beat rapidly? Does it feel like there's an acid pit bubbling in your stomach?

If you answer yes, you may want to check your caffeine intake.

It could be on overload.

Nutrition experts recommend teens limit daily caffeine intake to no more than 100 milligrams a day. It's the amount in one cup of drip coffee or two 12-ounce colas.

While a little caffeine may help you concentrate, fight fatigue, feel alert and even enhance endurance, when you consume too much you can be left with the jitters (and the agitation, headaches, insomnia and other not-so-pleasant effects of too much caffeine).[41]

So, if you do choose to consume products with caffeine, find your Goldilocks' balance: Consume enough, but not too much.

■ ■ ■

To Do: Limit caffeine intake to 100 milligrams daily.

How to wean from the bean

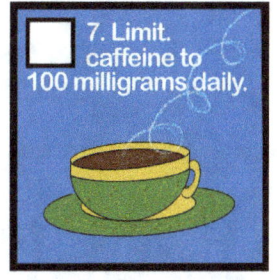

Reducing your caffeine intake too quickly can lead to caffeine withdrawal and its unpleasant side effects including headaches, fatigue, irritability and a loss of mental focus.

You can avoid symptoms of caffeine withdrawal by slowly cutting back on your daily intake over the course of one or two weeks. It's a better strategy than cutting back all at once, one that helps you comfortably wean from the bean.

Be sure to identify all sources of caffeine in your day. The usual suspects are coffee and other caffeinated beverages, energy drinks and shots, and chocolate foods and beverages. But, don't overlook less familiar sources like over-the-counter medications and dietary supplements.

When your daily caffeine intake drops to below the 100-milligram mark, you should be able to go cold turkey without experiencing any withdrawal effects.

If you want to know where caffeine could be hiding in your diet, check out **Caffeine by the Numbers** on page 124.

Notes:

> **8** For better test scores, fine-tune how you eat.

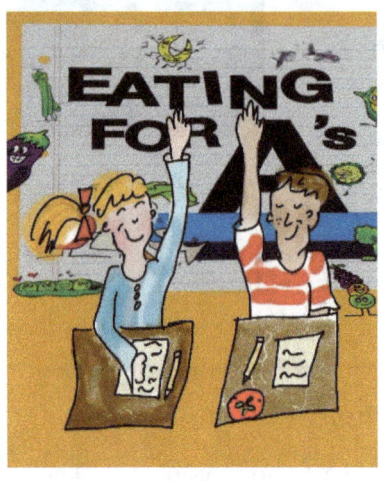

Eating healthy foods fills your body with energy and nutrients. Imagine your cells smiling back at you and saying: Thank you.
—Karen Salmansohn

What you choose to eat plays a key role in your academic success (or failure). Studies that look at the impact of diet on academic success have typically focused on eating breakfast or simply eating a well-balanced diet. The problem is these loosey-goosey endpoints fail to tell us much about specific food choices.

Now, a more focused approach has shed light on the foods you'll want to add to your daily plate, and the ones you'll want to avoid. In one study,[42] researchers investigated the link between diet and academic behavior in teens and children from the Australian Twin Registry (about 1,000 teens and kids up to 9th grade). When they crunched the numbers, the researchers found four specific food choices linked to better test scores: eating more vegetables, eating more fruits, eating breakfast and drinking fewer servings of sugary beverages.

■ ■ ■

To Do: Drink water instead of sugary drinks this week.

Are you eating for A's?

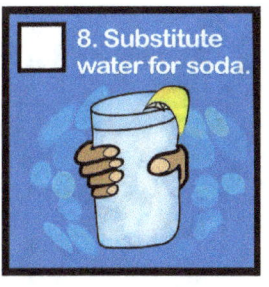

Four specific food choices have been linked to better test scores for certain academic skills. How many can you check off?

1 Eat more fruit. Eating more fruit (two or more servings per day) is linked to significantly better writing scores.

2 Eat more veggies. Compared to fewer times a week, eating vegetables at dinner every night is linked to significantly better spelling and writing test scores.

3 Eat breakfast. Eating breakfast every morning is linked to better writing scores.

4 Limit sugary drinks. Limiting the number of servings of soda and other sugar-sweetened beverages to less than one per day is linked to significantly higher test scores in four key skill sets: reading, writing, grammar/punctuation and math.

Interestingly, of all these food choices, the strongest predictor of academic success is limiting sugary drinks, so it's a great place to start if you want to fine-tune your diet for success in the classroom.

Notes: _____
_____
_____

9 For strong immunity, start with what you eat.

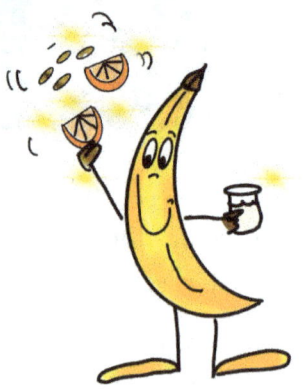

Your best defense against a cold, flu or other respiratory virus is a strong immune system. It's important because an achy body and a fuzzy brain can spell trouble, especially when you need sharp focus for a classroom project, sports competition or extracurricular activity.

Hope, purpose and determination are not merely mental states. They have electrochemical connections that affect the immune system.
—Norman Cousins

The good news is your ability to fortify your immune defense is hiding in plain sight in the foods you eat. Think vitamins A, B6, C, D and E and the mineral zinc.

This nutrient team works to activate natural killer cells and other immune cells, promotes a healthy inflammatory response and even helps maintain the protective membranes that line your nose, mouth, throat and intestinal tract.

In other words, when you choose the right foods, you can help fortify your immune defense.

■ ■ ■

To Do: Every day, eat one or more immune-fortifying foods, and supplement to fill any gaps.

5 foods for immune health

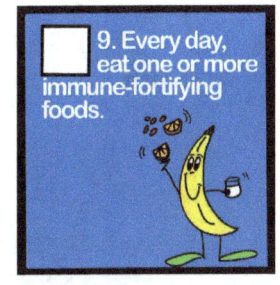

An active lifestyle needs serious immune health support, day in and day out. Making sure your daily menu is filled with foods with nutrients that fortify your immune function can help. Here are a few ideas to get started:

- **Almonds.** One serving (about 24 nuts) is an excellent source of vitamin E, providing about 40% of the Daily Value (DV). Other good sources of vitamin E include sunflower seeds and avocados.
- **Banana.** One medium banana is rich in vitamin B6 (20% DV). Other good sources of vitamin B6 include salmon, chicken breast and fortified tofu.
- **Beans.** One serving of cooked beans (½ cup) is high in zinc (26% DV). Other good sources of zinc include beef, poultry and lentils.
- **Low-fat milk.** A one-cup serving of milk is high in vitamin A (30% DV) and a good source of vitamin D (10% DV).
- **Citrus fruits.** One medium orange is an excellent source of vitamin C (130% DV).

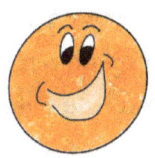

Notes:

10 — To fully enjoy your winter adventures, fortify your immune health.

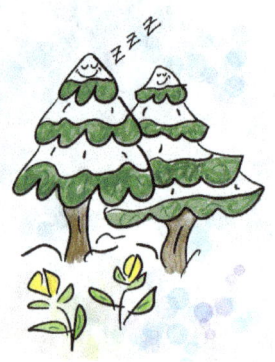

I wonder if the snow loves the trees and fields, that it kisses them so gently? And then covers them up snug, with a white quilt; and perhaps it says, Go to sleep, darlings, till the summer comes again.
—Lewis Carroll

During the winter (aka cold and flu season), viruses take flight, fill the air in crowded indoor spaces, and travel on shared surfaces.

No one wants these nasty bugs ruining their winter adventures. Eating more probiotic-rich foods like yogurt, sauerkraut, kimchi and other fermented foods can help. These foods contain friendly bacteria that temporarily take up residence in your intestine, where they block harmful bacteria from taking hold. That's good news since your gut is your body's first line of immune defense.

Proper hand washing also helps. Cold and flu viruses are often shared through hand contact, so making this a habit is an effective way to keep germs at bay. Don't forget to get restful sleep on a regular basis. Without it, your body's natural immune defenses are down. Get enough, and you're on your way to a stronger immune system.

■ ■ ■

To Do: Eat a probiotic-rich food at least three times each week.

Fortify your immune defense

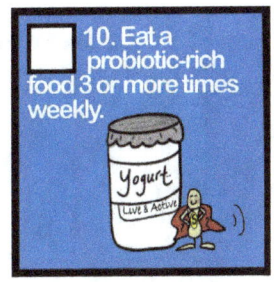

Habits that fortify your immune function don't need to be complicated. Here are a few simple habits that deliver serious immune protection:

- **Consume probiotics.** Consume foods or supplements that contain *L. acidophilus*, *B. bifidus* or other protective probiotics a few times each week or, preferably, every day. One popular food choice is yogurt, but only if it contains "live and active cultures." Other probiotic-rich foods include kefir, kimchi, kombucha, miso, natto, sauerkraut, tempeh and tofu.

- **Rub a dub dub.** Wash your hands using warm, soapy water. Be sure to lather up for at least 30 seconds before rinsing so you can get the most germ-busting benefits every time you wash.

- **Snooze.** Get about 9 hours of restful sleep each night.

- **Others.** Stay hydrated, reduce stress and get regular, moderate exercise.

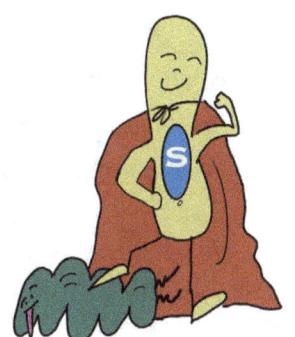

Notes:

11. To be healthier, happier and more successful, try the mealtime secret.

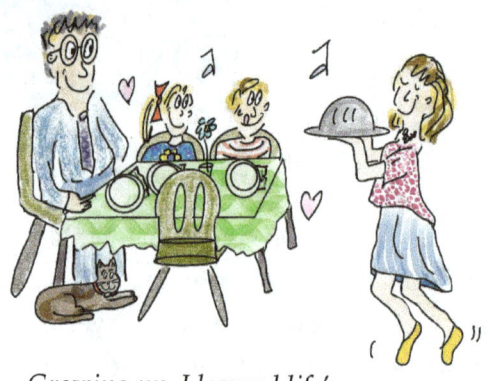

Eating a few meals each week with your family is one habit that can help you be healthier, happier and more well-adjusted, says over a decade of research.

Growing up, I learned life's important lessons at the dinner table.
—*Chef John Besh*

Do this, and you're also likely to get better grades in school and even maintain a healthier body weight than your meal-skipping friends.

So, what's the mealtime secret? It's not the food on your plate (no matter how nutritious), rather, it's the quality of your conversations.

In other words, it doesn't matter what you eat at a family meal (or where you eat, for that matter). What matters is you enjoy interesting, encouraging and upbeat conversations.

■ ■ ■

To Do: Eat at least five family meals weekly.

The mealtime secret for healthy weight

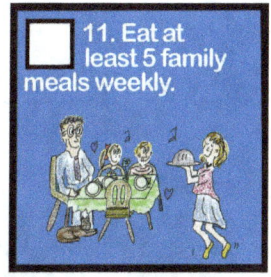

If you're working on losing excess weight, eating more family meals with upbeat conversations can help. In fact, researchers point to four types of mealtime talk that support a teen's weight loss journey:[43]

- Conversations that encourage everyone to share information in a clear and direct way.

- Conversations that encourage everyone to express their feelings.

- Conversations that encourage everyone to show genuine concern and interest.

- Conversations that encourage meaningful interactions.

Aim for at least five family meals each week. For example, gather for a family breakfast on weekend mornings and a few dinner meals during the week.

Remember, it doesn't matter what the meal is or where you eat it, as long as you're together sharing encouraging conversations.

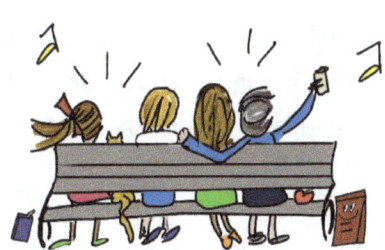

Notes:

12 To lower your pesticide burden, choose cleaner vegetables and fruits.

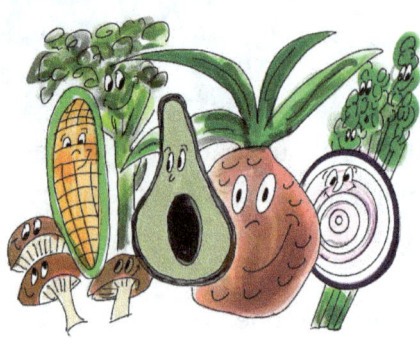

But man is a part of nature, and his war against nature is inevitably a war against himself.
—Rachel Carson

One of the most important food choices you can make to be your best you is to eat plenty of veggies and fruits.

Go ahead, crunch on an apple, dig into a salad or slurp away on your favorite green smoothie. But first, choose wisely.

Here's why. Your diet is the main source of pesticide exposure, and it's higher when you eat certain conventionally grown produce that rely heavily on the use of pesticides to kill bugs. The trouble is, pesticides remain in these foods, leaving them contaminated. Worse, some veggies and fruits are particularly good at retaining these caustic chemicals.

The good news is there's a simple way to reduce the pesticide load in your body: Choose organically grown veggies and fruits whenever you can.

■ ■ ■

To Do: Choose veggies and fruits with lower pesticide residue.

A cleaner way to eat

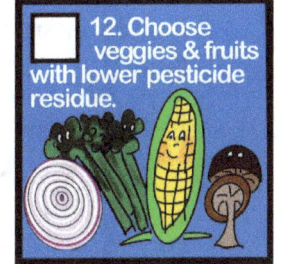

Each year, the nonprofit Environmental Working Group (www.ewg.org) publishes a guide that ranks conventionally grown produce based on pesticide contamination. Use this handy resource to help keep pesticides off your plate and out of your body.

The 15 "Dirtiest" Veggies and Fruits

This list ranks the 15 conventionally grown veggies and fruits with the highest pesticide contamination (the dirtiest ones). For 2022, the ranking is strawberries, spinach, kale, collard and mustard greens, nectarines, apples, grapes, bell and hot peppers, cherries, peaches, pears, celery and tomatoes. (For these foods, it's best to choose organic varieties).

The 15 "Cleanest" Veggies and Fruits

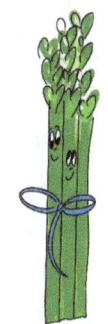

This list ranks the 15 conventionally grown fruits and veggies with the lowest pesticide contamination (the cleanest ones). For 2022, the ranking is avocados, sweet corn, pineapple, onions, papaya, sweet peas (frozen), asparagus, honeydew melon, kiwi, cabbage, mushrooms, cantaloupe, mangoes, watermelon and sweet potatoes.

Notes:

13   For an easier way to shape new habits, be like bamboo.

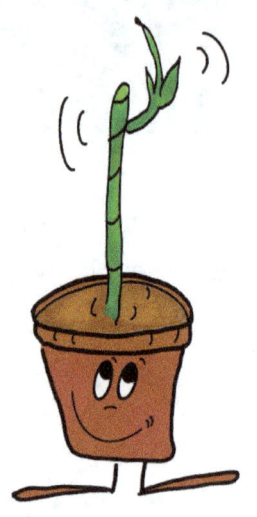

A journey of a thousand miles begins with a single step.

—Lao Tzu

If you're looking for a way to establish new healthy habits more easily (and make sure you keep them), be like the bamboo plant. The tiny bamboo seed takes about four years to break ground and form a little shoot. During the fifth year, however, it can grow a whopping 80 feet.

Turning new behaviors into solid habits occurs in the same way. It starts slowly when you consistently make minor changes in the behaviors you want to improve. Maybe it's drinking water rather than soda, planning your homework time better, taking time to unwind. You get the idea. The key is to pick something that resonates with you. Keep it up and, over time, all the little changes you make become regular habits that snowball into a powerful force that all but guarantees your new habits will last a lifetime. Making lifestyle changes can feel tough, but it doesn't have to be. You can make it easier by being like the bamboo.

■ ■ ■

To Do: This week, tweak one diet or lifestyle habit for the better.

Set SMART goals

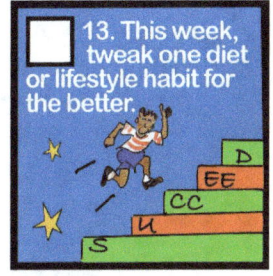

One of the best ways to make changes in your diet or lifestyle habits is to set SMART goals and track your progress.

SMART is an acronym for the five key elements of any effective goal. It stands for **S**pecific, **M**easurable, **A**ttainable, **R**ealistic and **T**imed. For example, the goal "I want to drink 8 cups of water every day for one week" is a SMART goal. Here's why:

- **Specific.** The goal aims to drink more water (rather than just beverages).

- **Measurable.** The goal aims to drink 8 cups of water per day (rather than just drink more water).

- **Attainable.** The goal is attainable because water is readily available.

- **Realistic.** The goal is neither too difficult (which can be frustrating), nor too easy (which can lead to boredom).

- **Time sensitive.** The goal has a deadline (one week), so you can evaluate your progress and adjust as needed. And, without a deadline, you may travel down the "I'll do it tomorrow" road to failure.

What SMART goal can you set and start tracking today?

Notes: _____
_____
_____

14 **Follow your taste buds, and your future self will thank you.**

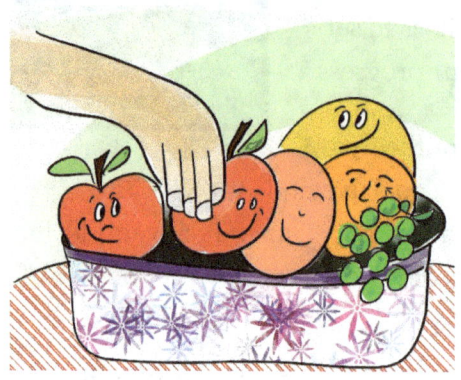

Change of habits are too light to be felt until they are too heavy to be broken.

— Warren Buffett

Can you predict whether you'll eat more veggies and fruits in your 20s, 30s and beyond? Yes, say nutrition researchers, and the reasons may surprise you.

In one study,[44] researchers followed 1,130 teens for 10 years. Each teen completed a food questionnaire and survey while they were teenagers, in their early 20s and, again, in their mid-to-late 20s.

After analyzing the data, the researchers found six key factors predicted a teen's future vegetable and fruit intake. Interestingly, one factor (taste preference) was directly linked to a higher intake of both vegetables and fruits.

In other words, now is the time to eat more veggies and fruits that tickle your taste buds. In this way, you're more likely to turn this delicious behavior into a solid habit that can nourish your body for years to come.

■ ■ ■

To Do: Try a new fruit or vegetable this week.

What's in your future?

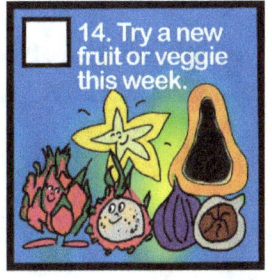

You can increase your odds of enjoying more vegetables and fruits as an adult when you have these six habits or beliefs in place during your teenage years:

- You like the taste (fruits and vegetables).
- You believe prep time will be fast (fruits only).
- You have plenty of choices at home (fruits only).
- You eat breakfast often (fruits only).
- You believe healthy eating offers health benefits (vegetables only).
- You snack less frequently (vegetables only). This one's a puzzle. It could be that when you snack less, you have a better appetite at mealtimes when veggies are likely to be served.

How did you rate? The more of these habits and beliefs you have during your teen years, the better.

Notes:
_____
_____
_____

15 To fill nutrient gaps, take a daily multivitamin.

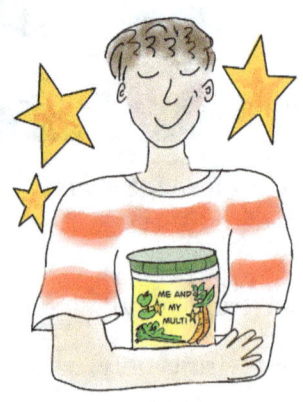

Before you decide to change your body, change your mind. Because, when your mind is ready, there is nothing that can stop your body.
—*Anonymous*

While a nutritious diet is the gold standard of healthful living, a busy life can get in the way of making the best food choices, day in and day out.

Not to worry, you can fill nutrient gaps by taking a daily multivitamin. It helps ensure an optimal intake of essential nutrients that tend to fall short in the teenage diet like vitamin A, beta-carotene, vitamin B12, calcium and iron.

A daily multi is especially beneficial for an overweight teen. Why? It provides antioxidants like vitamins A, C and E and the minerals selenium and zinc. This is important because excess fat cells can increase the production of harmful free radicals and oxidative stress. Antioxidants help neutralize this action and protect cells and tissues from damage.

■ ■ ■

To Do: Take a daily multivitamin.

Choose the right multivitamin

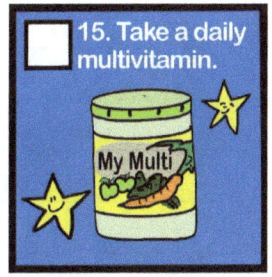

It's easier to find a quality multivitamin that meets your individual needs by starting with the basics:

1 **Choose a broad-spectrum multivitamin.** In this way, you'll get most (if not all) of the 20-plus essential vitamins and essential minerals for health. If a supplement contains an essential vitamin or mineral, you'll find it listed on the label with its percent Daily Value (%DV).

2 **Choose a multivitamin with key antioxidant nutrients.** Be sure your choice includes key antioxidant nutrients like vitamins A, C and E and the minerals zinc and selenium.

3 **Choose a multivitamin that includes phytonutrients.** In addition to essential vitamins and minerals, many quality multis provide phytonutrients such as beta-carotene, lutein, lycopene and others with health-promoting actions (including antioxidant activity).

Notes: _____
_____
_____

Notes:

Nutrition Resources & Quick Meal Ideas

Stretch Your gRAINBOW

When it rains look for rainbows, when it's dark look for stars.

—Oscar Wilde

Grains can add color to your meals and deliver the nutrients your active body and brain need.

Some colorful grains are listed below with more details on the next few pages, including what they look like, how they taste and, most importantly, how you can add them to your regular menu. (Follow recipe or package directions for cooking instructions.)

- Barley
- Brown Rice*
- Buckwheat Groats
- Bulgur
- Chinese Black Rice*
- Couscous
- Farro
- Himalayan Red Rice*

- Millet*
- Popcorn*
- Purple Thai Rice*
- Quinoa*
- Red Amaranth*
- Sorghum*
- Spelt (Wheat) Berries
- Teff*

* Gluten-free

Barley

With a pasta-like consistency, this chewy grain takes on the flavor of other ingredients, so it's a great choice for soups. Plus, barley is rich in beta-glucan, a type of dietary fiber that helps maintain healthy blood cholesterol, so it's good for your heart health too.

Brown Rice

Unlike white rice, brown rice contains both the bran and the germ, so it's more nutrient-dense, chewier and more flavorful. Its mild, nutty flavor and hearty texture make it ideal for soups, salads, side dishes and entrees.

Buckwheat Groats

Buckwheat groats are from grain-like seeds, so technically they are not a true grain. They are, however, a great source of prebiotics that promote the health of your digestive system. The fluffy, creamy texture and rich, nutty flavor make for one tasty hot breakfast, especially when you add a few nuts and raisins.

Bulgur

Made from cracked wheat, bulgur is commonly found in tabouli. It's a nutrient powerhouse that's packed with fiber, iron, magnesium and zinc, so it makes any dish better for your body and brain.

Chinese Black Rice

Cook this rice and watch its deep black color transform into a beautiful dark purple, thanks to anthocyanins. (The same powerful antioxidants found in eggplant, blueberries and other purple plant foods.) It has a nutty texture like brown rice, but a more earthy, intense flavor.

Couscous

A staple of North African cuisine, couscous is made from semolina flour. It's bland tasting on its own, but when combined with other foods, it soaks in all the flavors. This makes couscous a versatile grain that pairs deliciously with meat, fish, veggies, legumes or even fruit.

Farro

Farro is common in Mediterranean cuisine. The word farro refers to three types of ancient wheat: einkorn (*farro piccolo*), emmer (*farro medio*) and spelt (*farro grande*). All of them have a nutty flavor. Farro is available in whole grain forms and processed (semi-pearled and pearled) forms.

While the whole grain form of farro has more fiber and nutrients (like niacin and zinc), it can be a bit tougher (soaking it overnight helps soften it up). Try it as a hot breakfast cereal or sprinkled on a salad.

Himalayan Red Rice

This wonderfully chewy Asian rice has a deep rosy red color and an earthy, nutty flavor, not to mention plenty of nutrients like iron, magnesium, manganese and zinc. Pair it with meat, fish or veggies, add it to a salad, or use it in a rice pilaf recipe. (For a colorful treat, combine red rice with white rice, but cook the two separately because red rice takes longer to cook.)

Millet

This tiny, pale-yellow grain is often used for bird seed, but millet is definitely not just for the birds. This tasty grain is rich in protective antioxidants and magnesium. Enjoy millet as a breakfast cereal, sandwich bread for lunch, or in a pilaf at dinner. You can even pop millet like corn for a snack.

Popcorn

Popcorn is a teen favorite best made from scratch because the pre-packaged microwave popcorn bags often contain hydrogenated oils, which can harm your brain cells. (Fun fact: The kernels pop because they contain a small amount of water. The water turns to steam when heated and, as the steam builds up pressure, the kernels explode and pop.)

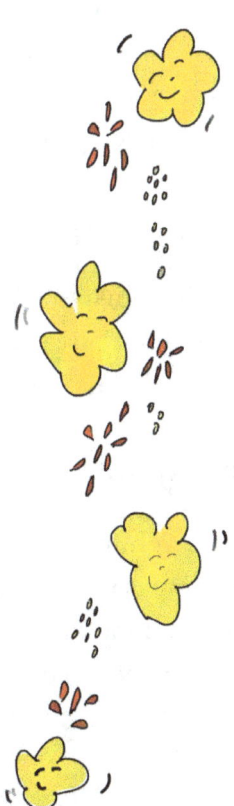

Purple Thai Rice

When you cook purple Thai rice, you're sure to marvel at its beautiful, shiny indigo color. This rice is traditionally used in desserts and other recipes with a sweet profile. To make sure your final dish looks great, cook the rice first (the purple color tends to bleed during cooking). Then, add other ingredients at the end of cooking.

Quinoa

Quinoa (pronounced KEEN-wa) is actually a seed that cooks like a grain. While it grows in several colors, white, red and black are the most common. The white variety tends to cook faster, while the red and black varieties are crunchier. All varieties have a similar nutrient profile and are a source of complete protein (all nine essential amino acids), which is rare for a plant-based protein food. Quinoa is ideal as a side dish to meats, seafood and veggies. You can even bake with it. Just look for quinoa flakes (similar to oatmeal flakes) or quinoa flour at your grocery store.

Red Amaranth

Red amaranth is another seed that cooks like a grain. It's one of the best whole grain sources of magnesium, an essential mineral critical for optimal muscle function.

Sorghum

Sorghum is a cereal grain that grows tall like corn. One variety is used to make sorghum molasses, a traditional sweet syrup popular in the southern United States. You can pop it like popcorn, cook it into risotto or add it to a lunch bowl.

Spelt (Wheat) Berries

Spelt is a type of farro wheat with a sweet, nutty, chewy goodness. It's not actually a berry, but a dark tan grain kernel that stays distinct when cooking. (For the best texture, soak them in water for an hour or longer before you cook them.) A one-cup serving of cooked spelt berries is an excellent source of muscle-building protein (over 10 grams) and hunger-curbing fiber (over 7 grams). Serve it up as a nutritious hot cereal topped with fresh fruit, a sprinkling of nuts and a dash of milk. Spelt berries are also a flavorful addition to salads and soups.

Teff

Teff is one of the smallest grains around, but it packs a nutritional wallop with over 120 milligrams of bone-building calcium per cooked cup. Plus, it has a creamy texture and a sweet, molasses-like flavor that is a delight for the taste buds.

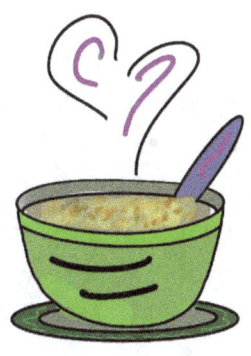

Carotenoid-rich Foods for Healthy Looking Skin

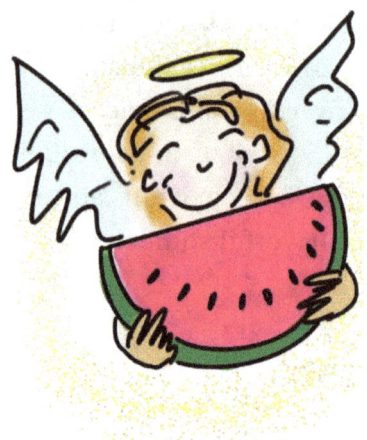

When one has tasted watermelon, he knows what the angels eat.
—Mark Twain

Fill your plate with foods that contain beta-carotene or lycopene. These are the carotenoids most likely to help give your skin a healthy glow.[45] For ideas, check out the good-better-best source list on the next page.

Plus, carotenoids serve as antioxidants throughout your body where they help neutralize harmful free radicals that form as a result of exercise, smoking, sun exposure, environmental pollutants, being overweight and other lifestyle factors.

It's an either/or thing. When carotenoids are used for their antioxidant action, they're unavailable to settle into your skin and provide a healthy appearance. This means you'll want to eat plenty of carotenoid-rich fruits and vegetables on a regular basis. In this way, you not only support your body's antioxidant needs, but you'll have plenty of carotenoids available for healthy looking skin. As always, choose fresh, local and organic produce, whenever possible.

Here's to putting your best face forward!

Beta-Carotene	Lycopene
Best Sources	
Carrots Spinach Sweet potato	Tomatoes and tomato-based foods like juice, soups, sauces, paste and purees. (Even ketchup is an excellent source of lycopene)
Better Sources	
Butternut squash Cantaloupe Greens (turnip, beet, chard, dandelion, collard) Lettuce (romaine) Mustard greens Pumpkin Sweet red peppers	Watermelon
Good Sources	
Apricots Broccoli Kale Lettuce (red leaf, green leaf, iceberg) Mangos Papayas Peaches (yellow) Peppers (sweet, green) Tomatoes and tomato products Winter squash (acorn) Yam	Grapefruit (pink, red) Papaya
Source: USDA FoodData Central (fdc.nal.usda.gov)	

Key Bone-building Nutrients

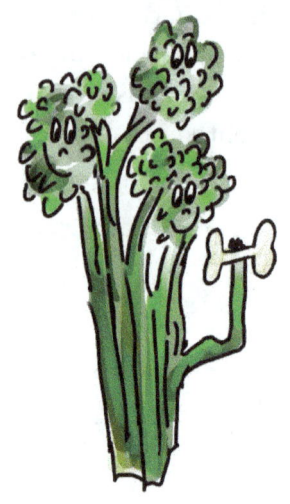

Let food be thy medicine.
—*Hippocrates*

Your bones need a wide range of nutrients for optimal growth and development.

You may be familiar with calcium and its role in bone health, but you may need a refresher on the other nutrients.

Here's a list of nine key vitamins and minerals you need to build (and maintain) strong bones, how they work in your body and what foods are good sources.

1. Calcium. This mineral provides structure to your bones (and teeth). Good food sources include dairy products (like milk and yogurt), dark green, leafy vegetables (like broccoli, kale and spinach), canned fish and beans.

2. Vitamin D. This vitamin helps your body absorb calcium. Good food sources include salmon and other fatty fish, egg yolk, cheese, mushrooms, milk and other fortified foods.

3. Vitamin K. This vitamin helps you make bone-forming proteins. Good food sources include green vegetables like collard greens, spinach, salad greens, broccoli, Brussels sprouts and cabbage).

4. Magnesium. This mineral supports calcium and bone metabolism, and bone cell function. Good food sources include plant foods such as dark green vegetables, seeds, nuts, legumes and whole grains. Other food sources include fish and milk.

5. Copper. This mineral is a building block for collagen (a key protein in connective tissues like bone and cartilage). Good food sources include seafood, nuts and seeds, legumes and whole grains.

6. Manganese. This mineral is an essential part of enzymes involved in bone metabolism. Good food sources include whole grains, nuts and legumes. Fruits and vegetables are moderate sources.

7. Zinc. This mineral is an essential part of enzymes involved in bone metabolism. Good food sources include meat, fish, poultry, milk and milk products. Legumes and whole grains are good plant sources, but they also contain plant phytates that can bind zinc and decrease its absorption.

8. Boron. This mineral may play a role in calcium and vitamin D metabolism. Good food sources include avocado, non-citrus fruits, peanuts and peanut butter, legumes and potatoes. In some areas, water can supply a significant source of boron.

9. Silicon. This mineral may play a role in collagen formation that's required for bone and connective tissue health. Good food sources include whole grains, especially oats, barley, rice bran and wheat bran.

Where's the Protein?

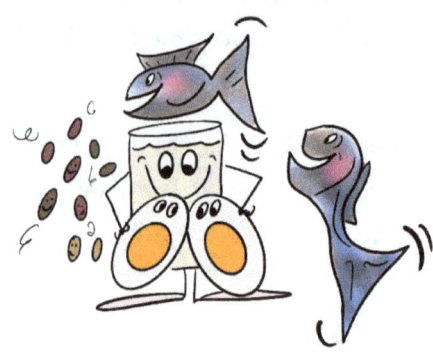

When life gives you lemons, you ask for something higher in protein.
—*Anonymous*

Two rules of thumb can help you estimate portion sizes of protein foods. First, a 3-ounce serving is about the size of a deck of cards. Second, a one-ounce serving is the size of a ping pong ball.

Remember, protein-rich foods can help you maximize the muscle-building benefits of resistance training, especially when you focus on the amount, type and timing.

- **Amount of protein.** Aim to consume about 90 grams of protein each day divided between your three main meals (at least 30 grams of protein per meal).

- **Type of protein.** Select protein-rich foods that provide about 2 to 3 grams of the amino acid leucine at each meal. This acts as a muscle-building trigger. (For food sources of leucine, see **Where's the Leucine?** on page 114.)

- **Timing of protein intake.** Eat a protein-rich meal within three hours of your weight-training workout to maximize its muscle-building actions.

Food Group	Protein Per Serving
Protein Powerhouses	
Chicken, fish, beef or pork (3 ounces cooked)	21 grams
Soybeans (½ cup cooked)	16 grams
Milk or yogurt (1 cup)	8 grams
Beans, black, garbanzo, kidney, lima, navy, pinto and white (½ cup cooked)	7 grams
Cheese (1 ounce)	
Cottage cheese (½ cup)	
Egg (1 large)	
Lentils, brown, green and yellow (½ cup cooked)	
Peas, blackeye and split peas (½ cup cooked)	
Peanut butter, almond butter, cashew butter and other nut butters spreads (2 tablespoons)	
Tofu (½ cup)	
Breads and Starchy Foods	
Ready-to-eat cereals (3/4 cup)	3 grams
Cooked cereals, pasta, rice (½ cup)	
Corn, potato or yams and other starchy veggies (½ cup)	
Bread (1 ounce; generally, 1 slice)	
Vegetables	
Carrots, broccoli, zucchini and other non-starchy veggies (1 cup raw, ½ cup cooked or ½ cup juice)	3 grams

Source: USDA FoodData Central (fdc.nal.usda.gov); Academy of Nutrition and Dietetics *Choose Your Foods* series.

Where's the Leucine?

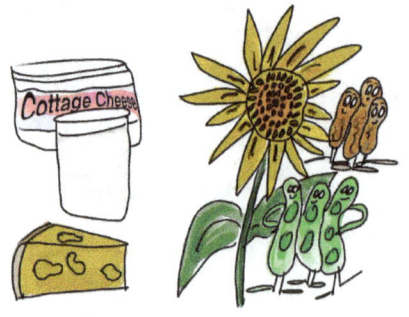

Nothing is impossible. The word itself says: I'm possible.
— *Audrey Hepburn*

Leucine is an amino acid found in a wide variety of protein-containing foods. For example, a 3-ounce serving of chicken provides 2.3 grams leucine. So does one cup of cooked soybeans.

You'll find the approximate leucine content in common foods (both plant and animal sources) on the next page, so you can more easily find foods that you like.

As you learned in **Look Good Tip #14**, you'll want to consume about 2 to 3 grams of leucine at each meal for optimal muscle building and toning benefits.

Food Group	Leucine Per Serving*
Plant-based Foods	
Tofu, firm (1 cup)	3.5 grams
Soybeans, cooked (1 cup)	2.3 grams
Navy beans, canned (1 cup)	1.7 grams
Lentils, cooked (1 cup)	1.3 grams
Beans (kidney, lima, pinto, white and others), cooked (1 cup)	1.3 grams
Split peas, cooked (1 cup)	1.2 grams
Chickpeas, cooked (1 cup)	1.0 grams
Oats, dry (1 cup)	0.8 grams
Teff, cooked (1 cup)	0.8 grams
Pumpkin seeds (1 ounce) Hemp seeds (3 tablespoons)	0.7 grams
Peanut butter (2 tablespoons)	0.5 grams
Peanuts, pistachios, sunflower seeds, walnuts (1 ounce)	0.5 grams
Almonds, cashews (1 ounce)	0.4 grams
Animal-based Foods	
Cottage cheese, low-fat (1 cup)	2.4 grams
Chicken breast, cooked (3 ounces)	2.3 grams
Pork chop, cooked (3 ounces)	2.2 grams
Protein powder, soy-based (1 scoop)	2.1 grams
Turkey meat, cooked (3 ounces)	2.0 grams
Beef, lean, cooked (3 ounces)	1.8 grams
Salmon, wild Atlantic, cooked (3 ounces)	1.8 grams
Tuna, canned (3 ounces)	1.6 grams
Yogurt, plain, low-fat (1 cup)	1.3 grams
Greek yogurt, plain, low-fat (7 ounces)	1.1 grams
Milk, low-fat (1 cup)	0.8 grams
Cheese (1 ounce)	0.7 grams

*Amounts are approximate.
Source: USDA FoodData Central (fdc.nal.usda.gov)

Where's the Fiber?

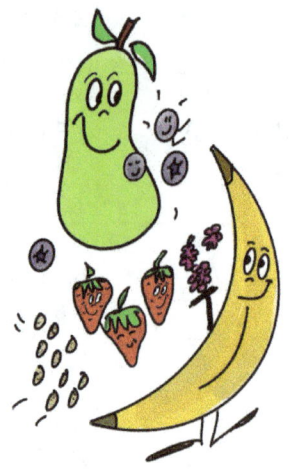

Every time you eat a fruit for the first time that year you need to make a wish.
—André Aciman

You'll find good to excellent sources of fiber listed in the table that follows as well as five simple ways to boost your intake below.

Remember, nutrition experts recommend that teens consume 14 grams of fiber for every 1,000 calories.

This translates into a fiber intake of about 26 grams per day for a teenage girl and 38 grams per day for a teenage boy.

1 Eat more dried beans and legumes. These fiber powerhouses are perfect for main dishes and side salads. Start with varieties that are easier to digest (and less gas producing) such as lentils, lima beans and split peas. You can also reduce the "toot" factor of any dried bean with a few pre-cooking tips. First, rinse the dried beans well and soak overnight in water. Next, drain the beans, cover with fresh water and cook until tender. Avoid adding salt, oil or spices until beans are tender, or they'll be tough. A one-cup serving (cooked) of dried beans or legumes provides about 10 to 19 grams of fiber.

2 **Eat whole fruits and vegetables; pass on juice.** The fiber reward here is huge. For example, when you munch on a crisp apple, you'll get 4 grams of fiber. Slurp apple juice instead, and you'll get less than 1 gram.

3 **Eat berries.** Berries are a sweet, fiber-rich treat. Plus, blueberries, strawberries and other berries have a natural sweetness that's especially ideal for desserts. A one-cup serving provides about 3 to 8 grams of fiber.

4 **Eat whole grain foods.** Foods made with whole grains (vs. refined grains) have more fiber. Brown rice, for example, has almost five times more fiber as white rice. So, choosing foods made with whole grains—bran, barley, bulgur, brown rice, popcorn, whole wheat pasta, wheat germ and others—rather than foods with refined grains can dramatically boost your daily fiber intake. A one-cup serving of brown rice or whole wheat pasta provides about 4 to 5 grams of fiber.

5 **Eat nuts and seeds.** These filling snacks make it that much easier to pass on chips, crackers, candy and other processed foods with little, if any, fiber. A one-ounce serving of nuts or seeds provides about 2 to 10 grams of fiber.

Food Group	Fiber Per Serving
Beans and Lentils	
Dried beans, cooked (1 cup)	11 to 19 grams
Lentils, cooked (1 cup)	16 grams
Split peas, cooked (1 cup)	16 grams
Baked beans (1 cup)	14 grams
Chickpeas, cooked (1 cup)	13 grams
Refried beans, canned (1 cup)	11 grams
Edamame (soybeans, boiled) (1 cup)	10 grams
Vegetables	
Squash (winter), cooked (1 cup)	9 to 10 grams
Sweet potato, cooked (1 cup)	8 grams
Artichoke, cooked (1 cup)	8 grams
Collards, cooked (1 cup)	8 grams
Pumpkin, canned (1 cup)	7 grams
Butternut squash, cooked (1 cup)	7 grams
Winter squash, cooked (1 cup)	6 grams
Peas, cooked (1 cup)	5 grams
Yam, cooked (1 cup)	5 grams
Kale, cooked (1 cup)	5 grams
Broccoli, cooked (1 cup)	5 grams
Fruits	
Avocado (1 medium)	9 grams
Berries, whole (1 cup)	3 to 8 grams
Pomegranate (1 cup)	7 grams
Pears (1 medium)	6 grams
Apple (1 medium)	4 grams
Oranges (1 medium)	3 grams
Banana (1 medium)	3 grams

Food Group	Fiber Per Serving
Grains and Pasta	
Bulgar, cooked (1 cup)	8 grams
Quinoa, cooked (1 cup)	5 grams
Whole wheat pasta, cooked (1 cup)	5 grams
Oatmeal, cooked (1 cup)	4 grams
Brown rice, cooked (1 cup)	4 grams
Nuts and Seeds	
Seeds (chia, flax, squash, pumpkin, sunflower) (1 ounce)	3 to 10 grams
Nuts (almonds, pistachios, walnuts) (1 ounce)	2 to 4 grams
Source: USDA FoodData Central (fdc.nal.usda.gov)	

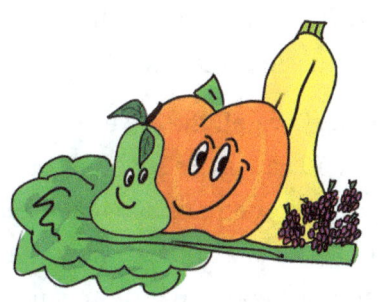

Power Smoothie Recipes

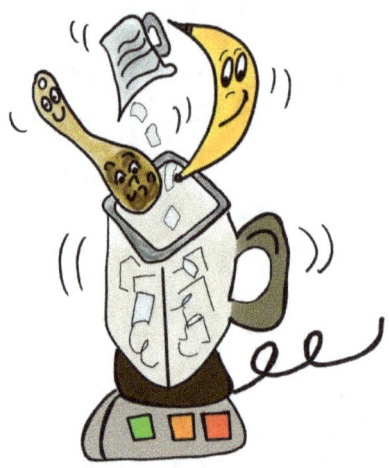

Mix a little foolishness with your serious plans. It is lovely to be silly at the right moment.
— Horace

Now that you know about how protein-rich foods promote more muscle building and toning benefits, you may be looking for a few easy recipes to boost your intake.

It doesn't get much easier than whipping up a smoothie.

Not just any smoothie, though. You'll want one that delivers a precise mix of protein (about 30 grams per serving) and the essential amino acid leucine (about 2 to 3 grams per serving) to fully stimulate muscle protein synthesis.

The recipes here check all the boxes with a few common ingredients. Plus, you can add a scoop of protein powder to help boost the leucine content of any smoothie. The exact amount of leucine will vary depending on the amount and type of protein powder you add, but in general, whey protein isolate powders have the highest leucine content followed by dry milk, casein, soy and pea protein powders.[46] To find the exact amount of leucine per serving, check the product label.

Peanut Butter Perfection Smoothie
(30 grams protein | 2.6 grams leucine)

Ingredients

2 cups chocolate milk, low-fat	(15 g protein | 1.4 g leucine)
1 banana, sliced and frozen	(1 g protein | 0.1 g leucine)
2 tablespoons peanut butter	(8 g protein | 0.6 g leucine)
1/3 cup rolled oats	(4 g protein | 0.3 g leucine)
1 tablespoon cottage cheese	(2 g protein | 0.2 g leucine)
1½ to 2 cups ice cubes	

Directions: Place all ingredients in a blender. Blend for one minute or until desired consistency. Enjoy!

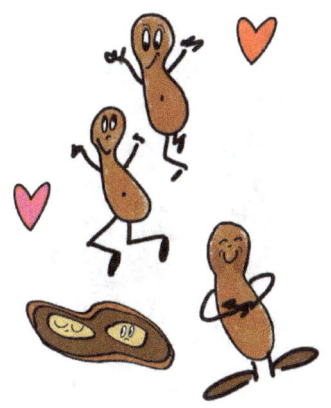

To me, peanut butter is the breakfast of champions!
—Greg Louganis

Yo' Berry Smoothie
(37 grams protein | 2.6 grams leucine)

Ingredients

1½ cups milk   (15 g protein | 1.4 g leucine)
6 ounces plain Greek yogurt   (19 g protein | 1 g leucine)
½ cup strawberries, frozen   (0.6 g protein | negligible leucine)
1 tablespoon cottage cheese   (2 g protein | 0.2 g leucine)
1 cup ice cubes

Optional: Add 1-2 teaspoons of honey for a sweeter flavor or substitute blueberries, raspberries or another berry for strawberries.

Directions: Place all ingredients in a blender. Blend for one minute or until desired consistency. Enjoy!

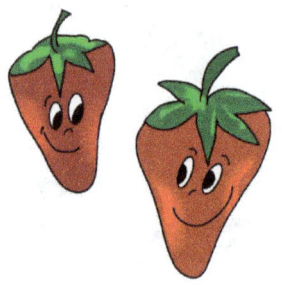

It is the sweet, simple things of life which are the real ones after all.
—Laura Ingalls Wilder

Banana Crunch Smoothie
(32 grams protein | 3.4 grams leucine)

Ingredients

1 cup low-fat milk	(10 g protein | 0.9 g leucine)
1 banana	(1 g protein | 0.1 g leucine)
1 scoop whey powder*	(18 g protein | 2.2 g leucine)
2 tablespoons almonds	(3 g protein | 0.2 g leucine)
1 cup ice cubes	

*1 scoop of whey protein powder is typically about 1 ounce.

Optional: Add 1-2 teaspoons of honey for a sweeter flavor

Directions: Place all ingredients, except almonds, in a blender. Blend for about one minute or until desired consistency. Add almonds, pulse blend for a few seconds so nuts are still a bit chunky. Enjoy!

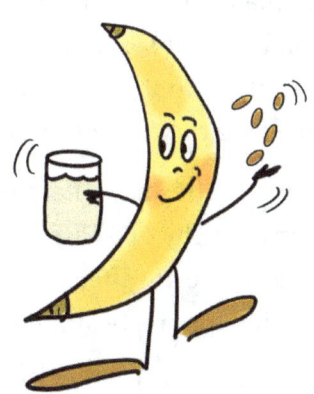

Always be ready when the time is ripe.
— Anonymous

Caffeine by the Numbers

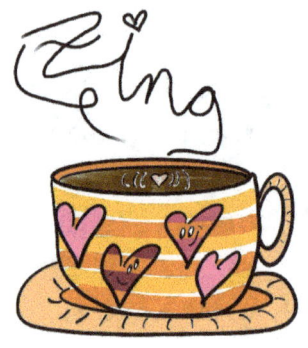

I love you a latte.
—Anonymous

As you learned in **Success Tip #7**, a little caffeine can have lots of benefits, but too much can make you feel anxious, irritable or worse.

For this reason, health experts recommend that teens consume no more than 100 milligrams per day.

You'll find common sources of caffeine listed on the next page like caffeinated beverages,[47,48] energy drinks and shots,[49] chocolate foods and beverages[50] and over-the-counter drugs and dietary supplements.[51]

Use this list to estimate your caffeine intake. Be sure to apply a little light math if your serving sizes are different from those listed. For example, a double shot expresso will give you twice the caffeine of a single shot (120 vs. 60 milligrams).

If you're looking for a refreshing alternative to avoid caffeine overload, consider chicory-based coffee substitutes. Chicory root is naturally free of caffeine. Plus, most of the fiber comes from inulin, so it supports healthy gut bacteria.

Herbal teas like passionflower, hibiscus, mint, rooibos and other caffeine-free varieties are another good alternative. From minty to bold to fruity and beyond, there's a flavor to delight just about anyone. Just look for "caffeine-free" on the label.

Food Group	Serving Size	Caffeine Content*
Coffee		
Regular, brewed	8 fl. oz.	120 mg
Ready-to-drink (bottled or canned)	8 fl. oz.	100 mg
Specialty (latte, mocha, cappuccino, Americano)	8 fl. oz.	95 mg
Espresso (single shot)	1 fl. oz.	60 mg
Carbonated Soft Drinks		
All types (cola, citrus and other flavors)	12 fl. oz.	55 mg
Tea		
Tea, yerba mate (brewed)	8 fl. oz.	125 mg
Tea, black (brewed)	8 fl. oz.	45 mg
Tea, instant powder	8 fl. oz.	30 mg
Tea, ready-to-drink, bottled	8 fl. oz.	25 mg
Tea, green (brewed)	8 fl. oz.	25 mg
Tea, white (brewed)	8 fl. oz.	15 mg
Energy Drinks/Shots		
Energy drinks	8 fl. oz.	180 mg
Energy shots	1 fl. oz.	65 mg
Chocolate Foods and Beverages		
Chocolate bar, sweet/dark	1 bar (1.45 oz.)	25 mg
Chocolate milk, hot cocoa	8 fl. oz.	about 5 mg
Chocolate ice cream, frozen yogurt, flavored yogurt	1 cup (135 grams)	about 5 mg
OTC Drugs/Supplements		
Caffeine-containing over-the-counter (OTC) drugs and dietary supplements	1 serving	up to 200 mg

* Amounts are approximate; mg indicates milligrams.

Breakfast in Under 5 Minutes

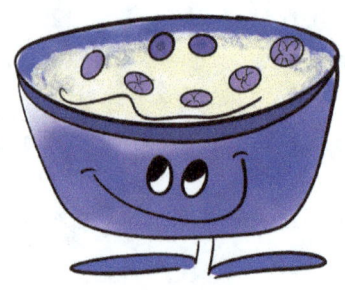

I'll eat some breakfast, then change the world.
　　—Hairspray soundtrack

That breakfast is the most important meal of the day isn't breaking news.

Not only does it break the long fast since your last meal the previous night, but breakfast gets you ready for the start of your new day.

Yet, breakfast may be the most underappreciated meal of the day, especially on school days.

On a good morning when homework is tucked into the backpack, hair and clothes fall into place, and there's time to spare, breakfast at the kitchen table gets half a chance.

On other days, those few morning minutes are precious. On mornings like these, a breakfast that can be made in less than 5 minutes can save your day. Need inspiration? Read on for five super-fast breakfast ideas.

1 **Cold cereal.** Pour a serving of cereal into a bowl, add milk and top with fruit or nuts, as desired. Choose a cereal that's a good source of fiber (at least 4 grams per serving) and low in added sugars (no more than 4 grams per serving).

2 **Hot cereal.** Scoop a serving of dry oatmeal into a microwave-safe bowl, add water (to totally soak the oats, but not so they're swimming), microwave for a minute. Add milk and top with sliced fruit, walnuts or raisins, as desired.

3 **Toast with a twist.** Toast two slices of bread. Spread with peanut butter or other nut butter and top with unsweetened applesauce. Microwave for 30 seconds.

4 **Microwave eggs.** Whisk two eggs and ¼ cup milk in a microwaveable dish. Microwave for 2 minutes. Add sliced mushrooms, peppers, broccoli or other veggie favorites. The eggs rise like a soufflé. Fluff with a fork and place back in the microwave for 30 seconds. Sprinkle with cheese. Enjoy!

5 **Yogurt parfait.** In a clear glass, add plain or vanilla yogurt, granola and your favorite fruit in alternating layers.

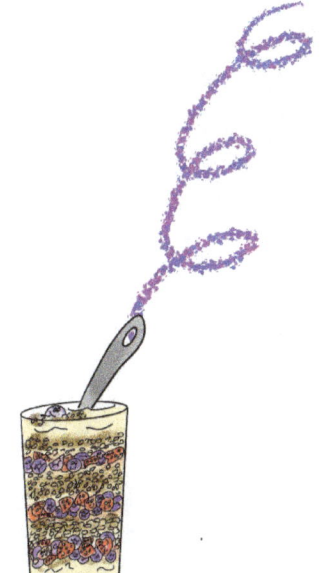

Acknowledgements

We owe a huge thanks to Katharine Noble, Liam Dunn, Maureen Dunn, Patty Crandall and the Williams clan (Brad, Andrew and Anika) for their thoughtful review and insightful comments. Thank you from the bottom of our hearts.

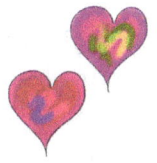

About the Authors

Lorna Williams, MPH, RD and Kathleen Dunn, MPH, RD are registered dietitians who have been collaborating on nutrition and health projects for over three decades. Along the way, Lorna has remained a big fan of a "make it fun" approach, while Kathleen gravitates to an "explain the why" approach. It's the perfect blend of whimsy and science to inspire people of all ages to take a nutrition-first approach to better living.

Lorna and Kathleen are members of the Academy of Nutrition and Dietetics. Lorna holds two bachelor degrees from the University of California, Berkeley, one in physiology and another in nutrition and food sciences, and a master's degree in public health nutrition from the University of California, Los Angeles (UCLA). Kathleen holds a bachelor's degree in biological sciences from the University of California, Irvine, and a master's degree in public health nutrition from UCLA.

References

15 Tips to Feel Good

1. Broussard JL, Ehrmann DA, Van Cauter E, Tasali E, Brady MJ. Impaired insulin signaling in human adipocytes after experimental sleep restriction: a randomized, crossover study. *Ann Intern Med.* 2012;157(8):549-557.

2. Matthews KA, Dahl RE, Owens JF, Lee L, Hall M. Sleep duration and insulin resistance in healthy black and white adolescents. *Sleep.* 2012;35(10):1353-1358.

3. Sleep Foundation. Teens and Sleep. Updated June 29, 2022. https://www.sleepfoundation.org/teens-and-sleep

4. Medina D, Ebben M, Milrad S, Atkinson B, Krieger AC. Adverse effects of daylight saving time on adolescents' sleep and vigilance. *J Clin Sleep Med.* 2015;11(8):879-884.

5. Sandhu A, Seth M, Gurm HS. Daylight savings time and myocardial infarction. *Open Heart.* 2014;1:e000019.

6. Noggle JJ, Steiner NJ, Minami T, Khalsa SB. Benefits of yoga for psychosocial well-being in a US high school curriculum: a preliminary randomized controlled trial. *J Dev Behav Pediatr.* 2012;33(3):193-201.

7. de Oliveira IJ, de Souza VV, Motta V, Da-Silva SL. Effects of oral vitamin c supplementation on anxiety in students: a double-blind, randomized, placebo-controlled trial. *Pak J Biol Sci.* 2015;18(1):11-18.

8. Lange SJ, Moore LV, Harris DM, et al. Percentage of adolescents meeting federal fruit and vegetable intake recommendations: youth risk behavior surveillance system, United States, 2017. *MMWR Morb Mortal Wkly Rep.* 2021;70(3):69-74.

9. U.S. Department of Agriculture and U.S. Department of Health and Human Services. *Dietary Guidelines for Americans, 2020-2025.* 9th ed. December 2020. https://www.dietaryguidelines.gov/

10. Hawton K, Ferriday D, Rogers P, et al. Slow down: behavioural and physiological effects of reducing eating rate. *Nutrients.* 2018;11(1):50.

11. Utter J, Denny S, Robinson E, Fleming T, Ameratunga S, Grant S. Family meals and the well-being of adolescents. *J Paediatr Child Health.* 2013;49(11):906-911.

12. Woolford SJ, Barr KL, Derry HA, et al. OMG do not say LOL: obese adolescents' perspectives on the content of text messages to enhance weight loss efforts. *Obesity.* 2011;19(12):2382-2387.

13. Schreier HM, Schonert-Reichl KA, Chen E. Effect of volunteering on risk factors for cardiovascular disease in adolescents: a randomized controlled trial. *JAMA Pediatr.* 2013;167(4):327-332.

14. van Woudenberg TJ, Bevelander KE, Burk WJ, Buijzen M. The reciprocal effects of physical activity and happiness in adolescents. *Int J Behav Nutr Phys Act.* 2020;17(1):147.

15. U.S. Department of Health and Human Services. *Physical Activity Guidelines for Americans,* 2nd ed. US Department of Health and Human Services; 2018.

16. Terry PC, Karageorghis CI, Curran ML, Martin OV, Parsons-Smith RL. Effects of music in exercise and sport: a meta-analytic review. *Psychol Bull.* 2020;146(2):91-117.

15 Tips to Look Good

17. Whitehead RD, Re D, Xiao D, Ozakinci G, Perrett DI. You are what you eat: within-subject increases in fruit and vegetable consumption confer beneficial skin-color changes. *PLoS One.* 2012;7(3):e32988.

18. Baldwin H, Tan J. Effects of diet on acne and its response to treatment [published correction appears in *Am J Clin Dermatol.* 2021;22(1):67]. *Am J Clin Dermatol.* 2021;22(1):55-65.

19. Camargo CA, Ganmaa D, Sidbury R, Erdenedelger Kh, Radnaakhand N, Khandsuren B. Randomized trial of vitamin D

supplementation for winter-related atopic dermatitis in children. *Atopic Derm Skin Dis*. 2014;134(4):831-885.

20. National Institutes of Health. Vitamin D Fact Sheet for Health Professionals. Accessed August 20, 2022. https://ods.od.nih.gov/factsheets/VitaminD-HealthProfessional/

21. Jung JY, Kwon HH, Hong JS, et al. Effect of dietary supplementation with omega-3 fatty acid and gamma-linolenic acid on acne vulgaris: a randomised, double-blind, controlled trial. *Acta Derm Venereol*. 2014;94(5):521-525.

22. Fitz-Gibbon S, Tomida S, Chiu B, et al. *Proprionibacterium acnes* strain populations in the human skin microbiome associated with acne. *J Investig Derm*. 2013;133:2152-2160.

23. Agak GW, Qin M, Nobe J, et al. Propionibacterium acnes induces an IL-17 response in acne vulgaris that is regulated by vitamin A and vitamin D. *J Invest Dermatol*. 2014;134(2):366-373.

24. Position of the Academy of Nutrition and Dietetics: Oral health and nutrition. *J Acad Nutr Dietetics*. 2013;113:693-701.

25. ALHumaid J, Bamashmous M. Meta-analysis on the effectiveness of xylitol in caries prevention. *J Int Soc Prev Community Dent*. 2022;12(2):133-138.

26. Jain P, Hall-May E, Golabek K, Agustin MZ. A comparison of sports and energy drinks: physiochemical properties and enamel dissolution. *Gen Dent*. 2012;60:190-197.

27. Cuddy AJC, Schultz SJ, Fosse NE. P-Curving a more comprehensive body of research on postural feedback reveals clear evidential value for power-posing effects: reply to Simmons and Simonsohn (2017). *Psychol Sci*. 2018;29(4):656-666.

28. Burd NA, Phillips SM. Protein and exercise. In: Karpinski C, Rosenbloom CA, eds. *Sports Nutrition: A Handbook for Professionals*, 9th ed. Academy of Nutrition and Dietetics; 2017:39-59.

29. Kerksick CM, Arent S, Schoenfeld BJ, et al. International Society of Sports Nutrition position stand: nutrient timing. *J Int Soc Sports Nutr*. 2017;14:33.

15 Tips to Succeed

30. Burton-Freeman B. Dietary fiber and energy regulation. *J Nutr.* 2000;130(suppl 2S):272S-275S.

31. Fatahi S, Matin SS, Sohouli MH, et al. Association of dietary fiber and depression symptom: a systematic review and meta-analysis of observational studies. *Complement Ther Med.* 2021;56:102621.

32. Dietary Reference Intakes (DRIs) Tables: Recommended Daily Allowance and Adequate Intake Values: Total Water and Macronutrients. In: Ross AC, Taylor CL, Yaktine AL, Del Valle HB, eds. *Dietary Reference Intakes for Calcium and Vitamin D.* National Academies Press; 2011. https://www.ncbi.nlm.nih.gov/books/NBK56068/table/summarytables.t4/?report=objectonly

33. Yang PJ, Pham J, Choo J, Hua DL. Duration of urination does not change with body size. *PNAS.* 2014;111(33):11932-11937.

34. Bujtor M. Can dietary intake protect against low-grade inflammation in children and adolescents? *Brain Behav Immun Health.* 2021;18:100369.

35. US Department of Agriculture, Agricultural Research Service. 2020. Food Patterns Equivalents Intakes from Food: Mean Amounts Consumed per Individual, What We Eat in America, NHANES 2017-2018. https://www.ars.usda.gov/nea/bhnrc/fs

36. Ng SW, Slining MM, Popkin BM. Use of caloric and noncaloric sweeteners in US consumer packaged foods, 2005-2009. *J Acad Nutr Diet.* 2012;112(11):1828-1834.

37. U.S. Department of Agriculture and U.S. Department of Health and Human Services. *Dietary Guidelines for Americans, 2020-2025.* 9th ed. December 2020. https://www.dietaryguidelines.gov/

38. Leidy HJ, Hoertel HA, Douglas SM, Higgins KA, Shafer RS. A high-protein breakfast prevents body fat gain, through reductions in daily intake and hunger, in "breakfast skipping" adolescents. *Obesity.* 2015;23(9):1761-1764.

39. Bauer LB, Reynolds LJ, Douglas SM, et al. A pilot study examining the effects of consuming a high-protein vs normal-protein breakfast on free-living glycemic control in overweight/obese "breakfast skipping" adolescents. *Int J Obes*. 2015;39(9):1421-1424.

40. Peña-Jorquera H, Campos-Núñez V, Sadarangani KP, Ferrari G, Jorquera-Aguilera C, Cristi-Montero C. Breakfast: a crucial meal for adolescents' cognitive performance according to their nutritional status: the Cogni-Action Project. *Nutrients*. 2021;13(4):1320.

41. Seifert SM, Schaechter JL, Hershorin ER, Lipshultz SE. Health effects of energy drinks on children, adolescents, and young adults. *Pediatrics*. 2011;127:511-528.

42. Burrows T, Goldman S, Olson RK, Byrne B, Coventry WL. Associations between selected dietary behaviours and academic achievement: a study of Australian school aged children. *Appetite*. 2017;116:372-380.

43. Berge JM, Jin SW, Hannan P, Neumark-Sztainer D. Structural and interpersonal characteristics of family meals: associations with adolescent body mass index and dietary patterns. *J Acad Nutr Diet*. 2013;113(6):816-822.

44. Larson N, Laska MN, Story M, Neumark-Sztainer D. Predictors of fruit and vegetable intake in young adulthood. *J Acad Nutr Diet*. 2012;112(8):1216-1222.

Nutrition Resources & Quick Meal Ideas

45. Whitehead RD, Re D, Xiao D, Ozakinci G, Perrett DI. You are what you eat: within-subject increases in fruit and vegetable consumption confer beneficial skin-color changes. *PLoS One*. 2012;7(3):e32988.

46. van Vliet S, Burd NA, van Loon LJ. The skeletal muscle anabolic response to plant- versus animal-based protein consumption. *J Nutr*. 2015;145(9):1981-1991.

47. Mitchell DC, Knight CA, Hockenberry J, Teplansky R, Hartman TJ. Beverage caffeine intakes in the U.S. *Food Chem Toxicol*. 2014;63:136-142.

48. Heck CI, de Mejia EG. Yerba Mate Tea (*Ilex paraguariensis*): a comprehensive review on chemistry, health implications, and technological considerations. *J Food Sci.* 2007;72(9):R138-R151.

49. Bill J, Gurley BJ, Kingston R, Thomas SL. Chapter 26: Caffeine-containing energy drinks/shots: safety, efficacy, and controversy. In: *Sustained Energy for Enhanced Human Functions and Activity.* Bagchi B., ed. Academy Press; 2017:423-445.

50. USDA FoodData Central. https://fdc.nal.usda.gov/

51. Gurley BJ, Steelman SC, Thomas SL. Multi-ingredient, caffeine-containing dietary supplements: history, safety, and efficacy. *Clin Ther.* 2015;37(2):275-301.

Index

Acne, tips for reducing
  borage oil, 44–45
  fish oil, 44–45
  low-GI foods, 40–41
  vitamin A, 46–47
Added sugars. *See* Sugar
Antioxidants, 98–99
  carotenoids, 38–39, 108–9
  definition, 4
Beta-carotene, 98–99
  food sources, 108–9
Bone-building nutrients, 56–59
  food sources, 110–11
  functions, 110–11
Borage oil. *See* GLA
Boron, 59, 111
Breakfast
  benefits of, 84–85
  benefits of high protein, 80–81
  fast and easy meal ideas, 126–27
Caffeine
  common sources, 124–25
  cutting back, 83
  intake guidelines, 82
  low-caffeine drink alternatives, 124
Calcium, 56–59, 98, 110
Carotenoids
  food sources, 108–9
  skin health, 38–39, 47
Citric acid, 52
Copper, 58–59, 111
Dental health
  chewing gum, 50–51, 53
  energy and sports drinks, 52–53
  protective habits, 48–53
DHA (Docohexaenoic acid), 44–45
Eating, benefits of slow, 28–29
Eczema, winter
  benefits of vitamin D, 42–43
Energy drinks
  caffeine content, 124–25
  stimulant effect, 7
  tooth decay, 52–53
EPA (Eicosapentaenoic acid), 44–45
Exercise
  music, 35
  recommended amount, 34
Eye health
  tips to enhance, 54–55
Fiber
  benefits of, 72
  food sources, 116–19
  recommended intake, 72, 116
  tips to determine adequate intake, 73
Fish oil. *See* EPA and DHA
Free radicals, 98, 108
  definition, 4
Fruits
  benefits of, 18, 84–85
  predictors of intake, 96–97
  ranked by pesticide residue, 93
  recommended intake, 19
  tips to boost intake, 18–21

GABA (gamma-aminobutyric acid), 14–15
GI (Glycemic Index)
　skin health, 40–41
GLA (gamma-linolenic acid), 44–45
Goal setting, 94–95
Grains
　adding variety, 26–27
　types of, 102–7
Gum, xylitol-containing, 50–51
Happiness, 34–35
Heart health
　beta-glucan, 103
　sleep habits, 8
　volunteering, 32
Hydration checklist, 75
Immune health
　foods for, 87
　nutrients for, 86
　tips to fortify, 88–89
Iron, 98
Leucine
　food sources, 64–65, 80, 114–15
　recommended amount for muscle building and toning, 64–65
Lutein, 54, 99
Lycopene, 39, 99
　food sources, 108–9
Magnesium, 58–59, 111
Manganese, 58–59, 111
Mealtime
　benefits of regularity, 90
　food portions, 70–71
　tips for great family meals, 91

Motivation and text messages, 30–31
Multivitamins. *See also* Supplementation
　benefits of, 98
　tips for choosing, 99
Muscle building and toning, 62–67
Oxidative stress, 98
Pesticides in plant foods, 92–93
Phytonutrients, 20–21
　definition, 4
Posture
　benefits of standing tall, 60
　tips to stand tall, 61
Probiotics, 88–89
Protein
　benefits of higher intake, 80–81
　food sources, 62–63, 81, 112–13
　leucine, 64–65
　powders, 65
　recipes (smoothies), 120–23
　recommended amount for muscle building and toning, 62–63
　timing of intake for muscle building and toning, 66–67
Recipes
　banana crunch smoothie, 123
　fast and easy breakfasts, 126–27
　peanut butter perfection smoothie, 121
　yo' berry smoothie, 122

Selenium, 98–99
Silicon, 59, 111
Skin health
    borage oil, 44–45
    carotenoids, 38–39, 47
    fish oil (DHA and EPA), 44–45
    GLA (gamma-linolenic acid), 44–45
    low-GI foods, 40–41
    vitamin A, 46–47
    vitamin D, 42–43
Sleep
    benefits of, 6, 8, 88
    recommended amounts, 7
    tips to enhance, 7, 9
Sports drinks
    tooth decay, 52–53
Stress reduction
    habits for, 10–11, 15
    vitamin C, 16–17
    yoga, 14–15
Sugar
    alcohols, 50
    tips to reduce, 52–53, 76–77
Supplementation
    bone-building nutrients, 56–59
    EPA and DHA, 44–45
    GLA (gamma-linolenic acid), 44–45
    immune health, 86–87
    multivitamins, 98–99
    probiotics, 89
    vitamin A, 46–47
    vitamin B6, 86–87
    vitamin C, 16, 86–87
    vitamin D, 42–43, 58–59
    vitamin E, 86–87
    zinc, 86–87
Teeth. *See* Dental health
Vegetables
    benefits of, 18, 84–85
    cruciferous, 24–25
    predictors of intake, 96–97
    ranked by pesticide residue, 93
    recommended intake, 19
    tips to boost, 18–25
Vision. *See* Eye health
Vitamin A, 46–47, 86–87, 98–99
    food sources, 47
Vitamin B12, 98
Vitamin B6, 15, 86–87
Vitamin C, 16–17, 86–87, 98–99
Vitamin D, 42–43, 58–59, 86–87, 110
Vitamin E, 86–87, 98–99
Vitamin K, 58–59
Volunteering
    benefits of, 32–33
Water
    benefits of, 74
    recommended intake, 74
    tips to determine adequate intake, 75
Weight management
    success habits, 91
Xylitol. *See* Gum
Yoga, 14–15
Zero period
    tips for success, 78–79
Zinc, 58–59, 86–87, 98–99, 111

www.ingramcontent.com/pod-product-compliance
Lightning Source LLC
Chambersburg PA
CBHW072047290426
44110CB00014B/1578